AF556438

AIDS and NGOs

INTERNATIONAL ENCYCLOPAEDIA OF AIDS- V

AIDS and NGOs

Editor
Dr. Digumarti Bhaskara Rao
M.Sc., M.A., M.A., M.Ed., Ph.D.
Reader & Research Director
R.V.R. College of Education
Srinivasa Nagar Colony
Guntur–522 006
(India)

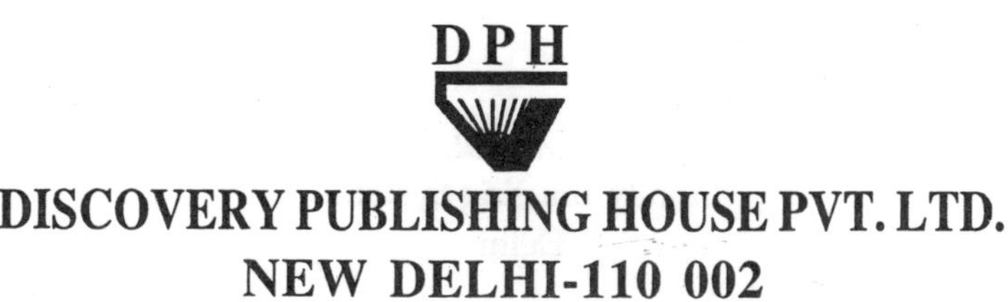

DISCOVERY PUBLISHING HOUSE PVT. LTD.
NEW DELHI-110 002

First Published – 2000
Reprinted – 2015

ISBN: 978-81-7141-527-4

AIDS and NGOs

Published by:
DISCOVERY PUBLISHING HOUSE PVT. LTD.
4383/4B, Ansari Road Darya Ganj
New Delhi - 110 002 (India)
Phone: +91-11-23279245, 43596064-65
Fax: +91-11-23253475
E-mail: discoverypublishinghouse@gmail.com
sales@discoverypublishinggroup.com
web: www.discoverypublishinggroup.com

Printed at:
Infinity Imaging Systems
Delhi

Preface

The HIV/AIDS is a new phenomenon in the human society. HIV destroys the immune system of human individuals, producing a defenselessness fatal state known as AIDS. The World Health Organisation has estimated that already one in every two hundred and fifty adults in the world is infected with Human Immunodeficiency Virus and according to WHO's projections a total of forty million men women and children worldwide will have been infected with HIV by the turn of this twentieth century. Visualising the devastating effects of the HIV/AIDS epidemic within our life times and beyond is difficult. Probably, no other disease in recent times has had the impact on human society generated by HIV/AIDS.

The HIV/AIDS epidemic has brought into focus many health related ethical, legal and human rights issues. This epidemic requires immediate and effective responses in new programming areas: attitudinal and behavioural changes, community-based care and support initiatives, and the maintenance of human development in the face of increasing rates of illness and deaths. At this point, education enters the scene as it can alter the HIV/AIDS situation since it brings change in the behaviour of the people.

This *International Encyclopaedia of AIDS* presents the worldwide information about HIV/AIDS, issues and challenges, reports and reviews, ethics laws and human rights, and educational activities and programmes to keep the policy makers, planners, professionals, activists, researchers, educationists, teachers and students well informed of the epidemic.

Dr. Digumarti Bhaskara Rao
26 January 1999
The Republic Day of India

Acknowledgement

I am thankful to the World Health Organisation and its associated offices for using their material namely School Health Education to prevent AIDS and STD: A Resource Package for Curriculum Planners-Handbook for Curriculum Planners. Student's Activities, Teachers' Guide, Global Programme on AIDS-HIV Prevention and Care: Teaching Modules for Nurses and Midwives, Global Programme on AIDS. Community HIV Prevention Handbook; STD care Management-workbooks 1-7, Facing the Challenge of HIV/ AIDS STDs: A Gender-based Response; HIV/AIDS and STD surveillance Data Management and Use-Report, Bangkok, 1995; Carrying out HIV Sentinal Surveillance-A Guide for Programme Managers, AIDS Prevention and Care in the workplace: Enhancing the Role of Private Sector; HIV Testing Policies and Guidelines; Carrying out HIV Sentinel surveillance; AIDS Prevention; Understanding and Living with AIDS; AIDS: A Modern Epidemic; HIV/AIDS in South-East Asia: IXth meeting of the National Programme Managers, New Delhi, 1993; Information, Education and Communication: A Guide for AIDS Programme Managers, Handbook on AIDS Home Care; HIV/AIDS in South-East Asia: A Pictorial summary; etc.

I am thankful to the United Nations Development Programme, UNDP's HIV and Development Programme, and UNDP's Regional Projects on HIV and Development for using their material namely Economic Implications of AIDS in Asia; Socio Economic Implications of the Epidemic; NGOs Working with Sex workers; NGO Responses to HIV/AIDS in Asia-Case Studies; HIV in the Workplace: Dealing with the Issues-Role Plays, Development and the HIV Epidemic, Law Ethics and HIV; HIV Law and Law Reform; Issue Papers; Study Papers; Working Papers; etc.

I am thankful to the Health and Nutrition Centre, Republic of Philippines for using its material namely sourcebook on HIV/AIDS

Prevention Education for Tertiary Educational Institutions.

I am thankful to the Curriculum Development Programme, Ministry of Education, Government of Thailand for using its material namely Institutional Modules for AIDS Education.

I am thankful to US Department of Health and Human Services: Whitman-Walker Clinic, Inc., USA; East-West Centre, USA; National AIDS Control Organisation, Government of India; Academy of Culture Communication Education Science and Service, Guntur, United Nations and its agencies for using their material.

I am grateful to Bhaskar Bhattacharji; V. Alexeev, Geeta Sethi, Elizabeth Reid, Mina Mauerstein-Bail, A. A. Trinidad, Palomi Cuchi, D. Pushpa Latha for their kind co-operation.

Dr. Digumarti Bhaskara Rao,
Secretary
ACCESS
D-43, S.V. N. Colony,
Guntur-522 006

Contents

Preface v
Acknowledgements vii

1. NGOs Working with Sex Workers 1
—Dr. A.J. Weeramunda
2. Sharing The Challenge of AIDS Prevention 68
—Jenny Huddart
3. Family Planning and AIDS Prevention 93
Jenny Huddart, Montu Pekanan
4. Commercial Blood Donors and AIDS Prevention 116
—Radium Bhattacharya, Jenny Huddart, Donna Bjerrgaard ,Glen William
5. Klong Toey: Facing Up to AIDS in a Bangkok Slum (Part I) 129
6. Klong Toey: Facing Up to AIDS in A Bangkok Slum (Part II) 145
—Glen Wiliams, Jinny Huddart, Karen Morita
7. Community Development and AIDS Prevention 155
—Jenny Huddart, Catherine Overholt
8. Marketing Ngo/Business Sector Partnerships 172
—James P. Reinnoldt
9. HIV in the Workplace 178
10. HIV: The legal Issues 182
11. HIV: Social Security and Insurance Schemes 186
—Prof. Nikom Chandravithun
12. Private Sector Collaboration on AIDS Prevention 188
—John Baker
13. Successful Partnerships: Action for AIDS-
Saatchi and Saatchi Advertising, Singapore 194
—Roy Chan, Bill Timmerman
14. Characteristics of Partnerships: The NGO Perspective 196
—Teresita Marie P. Bagasao
15. Characteristics of Partnerships: The Business Perspective 202
—Bill Timmerman

1

NGOs Working with Sex Workers

A.J. WEERAMUNDA
Department of Sociology University of Colombo, Sri Lanka

I. INTRODUCTION

The objective of this report is to describe and analyse the various strategies and approaches adopted by several non-governmental organizations (NGOs) in four Asian countries—India, Malaysia, Thailand and Sri Lanka—to control the spread of HIV/AIDS among sex workers. The study, sponsored by the UNDP, has great relevance in view of the general impression that Asian countries will become the new epicenter of AIDS.

Even though targeting of specific groups is an unhealthy practice, sex workers feature prominently in the above prognosis. A survey conducted in 1990 found that 75 per cent of Thai men had sex with prostitutes, almost half of them before they were 18. Government officials estimate that there are around 800,000 prostitutes in Thailand. Mostly aged between 12 and 16, twenty to thirty per cent of them are already HIV-infected. In northern Thailand, the rate is 44 per cent. A similar situation prevails in India where the level of HIV infection among Bombay's population of 100,000 to 500,000 prostitutes has jumped from one per cent in 1987 to 30 per cent in 1990.

In view of such astronomical number of sex workers existing in the developing world, combined with relatively higher rates of poverty and illiteracy, and oppressive social attitudes to prostitution itself, the task faced by NGOs becomes a rather colossal one.

Field work was undertaken by the author during a two month period (May to June 1994) during which a total of nine such organizations were visited. Research methods primarily consisted of interviews with staff working at various organizational levels, and observations conducted in certain "red light" areas.

The specific issues to be addressed through this study were:

1. How do NGOs create/build trust among sex workers?
2. What efforts are made to supplant or support self-help and other initiatives among sex workers?
3. How feasible is "safe sex" among commercial sex workers?
4. What are the linkages between commercial sex, transport corridors, poverty, etc, and the spread of HIV?
5. What legal/ethical issues are found in providing services such as counselling, promotion of condoms, and caring for sex workers who are HIV positive?
6. What specific projects are suitable for further documentation.

II. PROFFLE OF NGOs SURVEYED

1. The INDIAN HEALTH ORGANIZATION (IHO) is located in a municipal school within the J.J. Hospital premises in Central Bombay, India. IHO began work in 1985 starting with public AIDS awareness campaigns. A mobile clinic for treatment of STD and the peer education programme began in 1989 and 1991, respectively. It has since established branches in Pune, Sangh, Miraj, Kohlapur, Latur, Delhi and Goa where programmes similar to those in Bombay are being implemented.

IHO receives funds from the Ford Foundation and InterAides. Donations given by the Indian public, and proceeds from the sale of T shirts and publications such as AIDS ASIA are other small sources of funds. A counselling project for HIV positive people was funded by HIVOS.

IHO staff includes a programme director, one counsellor, an AIDS educator, three social workers, two doctors, two technicians, one administrator, an artist cum playwright, and two minor staff.

2. The GUJARAT AIDS PREVENTION (GAP), situated in the Siddha Chakka Apartments, Ahmedabad city, Gujarat, India, is a branch of the International Society for Research on Civilization Diseases and on Environment (SIRMCE) and mainly receives funding from CEBEMO (Holland). It provides AIDS awareness and education programmes particularly in Ahmedabad,

Mehsana, Valsad, Somnal and the tribal areas in Kutch. It also conducts free HIV testing, STD counselling, and a self-employment project for commercial blood donors. It publishes a newsletter in Gujarati and develops posters, pamphlets and booklets on HIV/AIDS. Recently it launched a safe sex education programme for truck drivers.

Principal sources of funds are CEBEMO (Holland), and International Planned Parenthood Association; with a budget of about four lakh rupees a year. Future plans include a mobile clinic and a library for sex workers of Surat, a creche for the children of sex workers, and adult and child education programmes in addition to work on HIV prevention in the red light areas of Surat. For the proposed activities GAP will need an additional 10 lakh rupees per year.

GAP staff includes a director, one psychologist, a doctor, one social worker, three counsellors, and 10 volunteer outreach workers.

3. COMMUNITY ACTION NETWORK (CAN) is situated in Virugambakkam on the outskirts of Madras city in Tamil Nadu, India has been operating since June 1992 with funds from the World Health Organisation (WHO), National AIDS Control Organisation (India), and the State AIDS Project Cell. It carries out target activities among sex workers and their clients; among circuits of men having sex with men; and with *Alis* (Transsexuals). It also runs a positive people's support group, STD care and services, and does networking with other NGOs.

The staff consists of a director, one programme manager, four social workers, one accountant, and 10 outreach workers.

4. SOUTH INDIA AIDS ACTION PROGRAMME (SIAAP), situated in Madras, was started in 1988 with funding from WHO and Ford Foundation, in partnership with the Panos Institute.

SIAAP's principal work is on STD/HIV focusing on long distance transport workers, women in prostituion and blind people. It has direct outreach programmes with all these groups in Tamil Nadu and runs similar programmes in partnership with other NGOs in the states of Karnataka, Andhra Pradesh and Kerala. Thus, NGO training and networking is a key activity in all southern states.

Other services include crisis intervention, pre and posttest counselling for STD and HIV, a hot line, supply of free food and support for HIV positive people in hospitals, networking with other NGOs in Tamil Nadu, and training their staff for HIV prevention. SIAAP is currently developing an AIDS information manual in braille for the visually handicapped.

The regular staff includes one director, three programme Managers, eight social workers, two counsellors, 15 outreach workers, a materials manager, one full-time and another part-time accountant, one full-time and another part-time secretary.

5. TENAGANITA, which in Malay means 'women's force', is located in downtown Kuala Lumpur and has been working on women's issues for many years. Specifically, it provides health care programmes and training for women working in plantations and factories. It also gives individual and family counselling and its office serves as a drop-in-center. In addition, it has ventured into areas such as HIV/AIDS education, providing legal aid for women, and maintains a 'half-way' house for sex workers, some of who are HIV positive.

The all-women staff includes a director, five social workers, three counsellors and one receptionist.

6. PINK TRIANGLE (PT) is a gay organization situated on the outskirts of Kuala Lumpur. It began AIDS prevention work among the city's gay population in 1987 with funding from AIDA and subsequently from NOVIB and HIVOS. Besides maintaining a hotline, the NGO has ventured into AIDS prevention among sex workers and maintains IKHLAS, a drop-in-center in Chowkit, a central part of the city which is host to a large number of sex workers and drug users. PT is currently engaged in setting up a PWA (People with AIDS) network for the Asia Pacific region.

The staff includes a director, one programme manager, one administrator, an officer in charge of human resources, and four outreach workers.

7. The THAI RED CROSS SOCIETY is situated in Bangkok and its AIDS unit is primarily engaged in research on sex workers including compilation and analysis of data from secondary sources, and maintaining a clinic for voluntary testing and counselling for STD. It is presently engaged in mapping all commercial sex establishments in Bangkok and all Thai provinces. It also conducts a multi-site intervention project in Thailand, Mexico, and Ethiopia.

The staff includes one director, three counsellors, and two office assistants.

8. EMPOWER, an acronym for "Empowerment Means Protection of Women Engaged in Recreation", began work in 1985 with support from the Ford Foundation, concentrated its efforts on promoting AIDS education among sex workers in Thailand. It has since expanded its activities to other areas such as providing basic education, language training, health counselling on STD and HIV, general counselling, and condom promotion among sex workers. The NGO operates through three outreach centers—two in Bangkok, and one in Chiang Mai—and a

resource center in the town of Nonthaburi. In addition, it has a positive people's support group called Naam Chewit, and Honey Bee Special which is a condom promotion show. All activities are undertaken by a staff of 15 persons including a director, one national coordinator, and eight international volunteers who are not permanent members.

9. ACCESS, which stands for "AIDS Counselling Centers and Counselling Services", was established in early 1991 and is located in Bangkok. Its AIDS prevention campaigns are targeted at the general population and also specific groups including sex workers. It maintains a hotline and provides counselling and support services for PWAs and their partners and/or families. Its principal geographic areas are Bangkok city and Northern Thailand. It has received funds from ICCO (Netherlands), MISERENOR (Germany), the Thai Ministry of Public health, AIDSCAP and NAPAC.

The staff includes one director, 12 staff assistants, 20 fulltime community workers, and five part-time telephone counsellors. Another 18 people work as unpaid telephone counsellors.

10. COMMUNITY FRONT FOR PREVENTION OF AIDS (CFPA) is a Sri Lankan NGO formed in 1992 by representatives of three service clubs, Lions, Kiwanis, and Rotary, and from other service organizations in the country. Its main office is situated at 1 20/ 20,Vidya Pedesa, off Wijerama Mawatha, Colombo 7. CFPA received funding from USAID to launch a safe sex campaign among sex workers in Sri lanka's Southern Province which has a large number of tourist resorts and establishments catering to the tourist industry. CFPA is the only Sri Lankan NGO concerned with HIV prevention among sex workers. It aims to undertake AIDS awareness campaigns and create local task forces throughout the island country.

CFPA's staff include an Administrator, a clerk/typist, and an accountant. Field staff for specific programme inputs are recruited on a short term contractual basis. For information on Sri Lanka, the author has relied on his own experiences while working from September 1993 to January 1995 as coordinator for an AIDS prevention programme among sex workers in a province of the Island; launched by a Sri Lankan NGO.

III. BACKGROUND OF THE STUDY

India

According to IHO, though as of March 1, 1994, only 710 full-blown AIDS cases and nearly 14,000 HIV carriers have been reported by over 80 surveillance centers of NACO (National AIDS Control

Organisation), the real figures could be alarming. IHO estimated two million HIV infections and 1,00,000 AIDS cases in India at the end of 1993 (Gilada 1994:3). By the year 2000, other factors remaining unchanged, IHO estimates 30-50 million HIV infected people in India. This means, five per cent of the population, and every tenth sexually active adult Indian will have been infected. India as a whole is ranked as a high prevalence country for STD with a rate of 5.1 per cent plus (Khan et al, 1991:5). Cited as a 'silent volcano', it is believed that within a few years India will be facing a problem similar to that of many African societies.

Bombay

IHO estimates over 150,000 HIV infections and 15,000 AIDS cases in the city of Bombay alone. Among regular hospital patients, TB patients, STD patients and healthy blood donors, HIV positivity is 12-15 per cent, 20 per cent, 25 per cent, and 1.6 per cent, respectively. Among commercial sex workers it is more than 50 per cent (Gilada, op.cit.). According to IHO, seven per cent of all blood tested at government hospitals is HIV positive. As Dr. Gilada puts it, "Even leaving a margin for possible error, this comes to a high number of people." Adding, "In one large brothel of 4000 prostitutes, eight out of 11 samples tested in 1993 were found to be positive. Each minute there are 10 customers visiting that building. From seven in the morning till ten in the night there are people coming for sex: married, unmarried, students with school bags, and teenagers. An estimated 75,000 married people visit the red light areas of Bombay every day and, if they get HIV, they will give it to their wives. Extramarital affairs are common in India, though hidden."

Dr. N from IHO, sees the problem in terms of STDs: "Out of an estimated 250 million cases of STD in the world, India has about 50 million making it the highest for any country. STD enhances chances of HIV infection by 15 per cent. And if we are number one for STD, we will naturally be number one for HIV. According to WHO, five per cent of the total Indian population will be HIV affected by the year 2000. Of every 10 people, one will be positive. Every day, 15,000 people will be dying."

The problem is complicated by hospital practices: "Some private hospitals unethically take blood from the patient without his or her knowledge for HIV testing. If found positive, the patient is discharged. Again, of five government hospitals in Bombay, only one admits full-blown AIDS cases. All the others admit patients only to discharge them in a day or two."

IHO identifies three levels of HIV incidence in Maharashtra, with levels highest in large cities such as Dhule, Sangli, Pune, and Satara. Smaller towns such as Sholapur, Nagpur and Nashik form the secondary level. Other towns in the state make up the tertiary level. All these urban centers are connected by rail and express highways. Truck stopovers are common places for small time prostitution with truck drivers and cleaners serving as the main clients: as also the 'carriers' of HIV transmission.

Those involved in sex work can be classified into three types based on the type of sex they engage in: (1) females for heterosexual sex (2) eunuchs and transvestites who have sex with men, and (3) males who have sex with males. Female sex workers come to Bombay from all over India, but more from the states of Karnataka, Andhra, Tamil Nadu and recently, from Nepal. Some also come from Madhya Pradesh, Uttar Pradesh, Rajasthan, Maharashtra, and West Bengal.

According to IHO, economic and institutional factors work together to widen the ranks of those entering the sex trade. As one official puts it, "Poverty is the underlying cause, but not the only cause. Even if someone is poor and you ask them to sleep with you, they will not agree to it. Victims of rape, incest, abduction, failed marriages, and temple prostitution are the main causes, combined with poverty. If someone is known as the daughter of a prostitute, who will want to marry her? Who will accept her into society? If someone is raped, who will accept or marry her? It is because she cannot survive that she runs away. However, if there was an economic alternative for her, like access to her share of parental property, or if she was educated, she would not get into prostitution but take up some other work. Nobody gets into prostitution voluntarily because of poverty. People look upon it as immoral work; a woman's chastity is like glass, which once broken cannot be put together. This idea is deeply ingrained in society".

According to IHO's Director, factors which combine with poverty account for a large majority of women entering sex work; while temple prostitution accounts for about a third of it. How temples are related to prostitution is given in the following account: "It is a system of concubinage through religion and power which exploits the lower classes of the community. A 'barren' woman without a child or delayed pregnancy will make a vow to dedicate the first child, whether male or female, to the Goddess *Yellamma (Kali,* as she is known in Maharashtra). The ceremony takes place when the child reaches seven or eight years of age. After that, the child goes back to live with her parents. On reaching puberty, she is taken to a temple where an auction takes place.

"The highest bidder gets to use the child sexually for the first time. In earlier times, the bidder also had to take care of the child for the rest of its life. With the decline of this system of patronage, and particularly when such children could not get a part of the family inheritance, the custom became a means of entering prostitution. Male children who are also dedicated to *Yellamma* are called jogappa. They are supposed to dress and even behave like girls and have sex with men. Like their female counterparts, the *devdasi,* they also get into prostitution. If a good break or good education comes by, they go into other areas such as singing or dancing. Since they are dedicated to the Goddess for the rest of their lives, they do not get married."

Prostitution takes place in large brothels in central Bombay where the owners or managers give the girls protection from police arrest in return for a portion of their earnings. Large brothels, having thousands of sex workers, are found in Kamathipura, Falkland Road, Pavala Street, and Grant Road in central Bombay. Brothels are also found near Hanuman Gali, Ghatkopar (along the railway line), Sonapur, Bhandup (on old Agra Highway), Sewri, Sion and Koliwada which are the suburbs of Bombay. The total number of female sex workers in Bombay is estimated to be between 100,000 and 150,000.

Kamathipura, for example, has 16 different lanes with a total population of 15,000 sex workers. Jumna Mansion alone has about 4000 girls in its five-storied structure. Krishan Building, a similar structure, has about 6000 girls. The area is full of-small business establishments catering to the daily needs of both sex workers as well as their clients. Estimated HIV incidence, according to IHO, is at least eight out of 11 sex workers in Jumna Mansion. The rate could actually be increasing since some sex workers treated for TB and STD are not responding to drugs.

General living conditions can be highlighted through a section of the author's field notes taken on a visit to Krishna Building: "The access lane is lined with low income housing on one side and shanties on the other. It is about 11.00 a.m. and people are reclining on beds made of bamboo frames and coir rope. Men, women, children and young adults squat on the ground, lounging or sleeping wherever there is space. The street is lined with garbage, scavenging rats, and rotting food as one walks towards its end."

An inside view of a large brothel on Falkland Street, from the field notes: "This brothel which is about four stories has a large dormitory-type building with one main entrance and has about 7,000 girls. It is about 10 in the morning. The main corridor is flanked by small rooms for the use of customers. It is crowded with about 50 girls standing, dressed up and waiting for customers. The area is roughly 120 square feet in size. Amidst the smell of perfume and talcum powder is a heap of rubbish containing used condoms, stacked against a corner of the waiting hall. In the rooms, used only for sex, girls are getting ready to meet customers. There is no furniture other than beds. The only signs of a home are found in the room occupied by the brothel manager, a woman of about 52 years, who works as a member of IHO's condom promotioncampaign.

The rooms are small and usually have a light and fan. They are not meant for lounging around or having long chats, but for quick sex which usually takes anything between five to 10 minutes."

Some sections of the brothel serve as living quarters as well. Female sex workers carry on their daily chores here including caring for their children, washing, cleaning, cooking, doing bead work, writing letters home, playing cards or watching TV in small groups. Old retired sex workers also assist in the daily work, and are paid a small amount of money for it. Vendors of various wares ply in and out of this maze of humanity—Itinerant book sellers, fortune tellers with parrots and cards, and men who are skilled in tattooing or cleaning ears with sharp, pointed instruments. The term "commercial sex" has therefore to be placed within the context of an active, urban slum community.

Dr. N of IHO is of the opinion that sex workers are the most exploited section of society. "Every month, a fixed amount of money goes as a bribe to the concerned police stations. If it is a big brothel, the payment is more, say, Rs 3,000 a month. If there are only 20 or 30 girls it is less. And if there are minor girls (under 13 or 14 years) the brothel has to pay even more. The asking rate is usually Rs 15 or less per customer. The sex workers take money before the sexual act begins; half of which goes to the brothel keeper. If the girl has seven or eight clients a day, she can make 60 or 70 rupees daily. But most of this is spent on food and medicine. Usually, the girls do not cook, buying food from outside.

"The supplier charges one or two rupees extra for their food. Even for medicines they are overcharged. If the price is, say, five rupees, they have to pay Rs 7.00 or Rs 7.50. At every step they are exploited. Loans given to sex workers by Pathan moneylenders are also at higher interest rates (10 per cent per month or more). In addition, if they contract STD, another 60 to 100 rupees have to be spent for a doctor. The streets are lined with quacks making matters even worse. If they do not use condoms and get STD, it means more and more visits to the doctor. And to top it all, they often have to send home money for dependents."

Bombay also has a *hijra* (male transvestite or eunuch) population of about 2,000 who engage in commercial sex with males. IHO estimates HIV positivity among them to be about 50 per cent. Beaches bordering the city are also used for commercial sex involving males. Ashok Row Kavi, editor of *Bombay Dost,* a gay magazine, estimates that there are about 800 males aged between 17 and 40 who work as masseurs for male clients visiting the beaches. Many of the masseurs also engage in oral and anal sex once the general public leaves the beach later in the evening. Many of these younger males live in small crowded rooms rented in the vicinity. Most of them are from the villages and have taken to the trade due to lack of any other employment.

Gujarat

According to GAP director, attention on HIV/AIDS was aroused by a newspaper article which said that out of a sample of 466 blood donors, 435 were found to be positive. That was four years ago. GAP was formed as a branch of SIRMCE in response to this reality. In Ahmedabad city, officially there are 329 HIV positive cases so far and 18 full-blown cases of AIDS. GAP's estimate is however around 1000 positive cases. In Surat, for example, where the red light district is located, in a particular clinic, two new cases of positive blood samples are found every month.

The GAP director sees a direct link between poverty and prostitution. "Unless and until that problem is solved all other problems will stay with us," she says. The city has had a large population of industrial workers mostly employed in the textile mills. During the last six years, with more and more mills closing down, there has been a steady rise in poverty, forcing some families into prostitution as a means of livelihood. For some unemployed youths donating blood has become a source of income.

According to GAP estimates Ahmedabad city has about 7000 sex workers, many of who operate individually, getting picked up at bus stops or railway stations; thus making it difficult to work among them. Surat has a red light area with about 700 sex workers coming from different states of India, and living in about 100 small brothels. About 50 of these are of Nepali origin. The demand for Nepalis is a result of inhibitions of Indian women who do not allow oral or anal sex. While Nepalis allow such practices, they charge more money for it. Because they earn more, they are also more prone to harassment by police, since many of them have entered the country illegally.

Surat also has a large influx of labourers who come without their families from the surrounding country side to work as construction labourers and gardeners. They form a large part of the clientele visiting Surat's red light area where almost all sex workers belong to the low income level.

In Surat the brothels are smaller in size compared to those in Bombay, but women have greater freedom to move in and out of them. Every establishment has between five to 15 women, operated by a woman who usually has a husband, or a steady boyfriend whom she calls husband. The operators often have links with their counterparts in Bombay and other cities, and even arrange for transfers from one city to another on a short term basis. According to GAP, the movement takes place because of the personal need to experience life in other cities. Sex workers also move out of one place once they are found to be HIV positive. This is to avoid stigmatization by other sex workers. One reason for staying in a brothel is to overcome the acute housing problem in Surat. NGO officials are not certain as to how many women are brought and kept by force, even though some are known to be forced into prostitution.

A large proportion of women in the trade are between 18 and 35 years of age. Quite a few are over 35 years and continue in the profession, ending up as servants and cleaners or as brothel operators. There are almost no cases where they drop out of prostitution altogether.

Madras

Unlike Bombay or Surat, there are no specified red light areas in Madras. When CAN began work among sex workers in late 1992, it had no idea of the extent and nature of prostitution in the city. With help from WHO and a foreign anthropologist, CAN did an ethnography in 1992—the only such exercise encountered in the course of the study—on the commercial sex trade and mapped the networks, circuits of different types of sex workers, and the possible numbers involved in each location. Through the survey, CAN had estimated the total population to be around 6000, of which nearly half were female sex workers. They are classified in terms of different modes of operation and gender as follows:

Female sex workers, numbering around 3000, are grouped into three categories:

(a) Family girls, numbering around 1800, operate completely underground. They usually live with an elderly couple posing as parents, but who actually manage the operation in an ordinary house, getting clients through female brokers called *aunties.* Some of them have also taken up part-time jobs in hospitals and offices which fetch them salaries of about six to eight hundred a month. Sex is their main source of income even though, very often, their family members or neighbours do not know anything of their occupation.

(b) Brothel girls number around four to five hundred with two to four girls per brothel. Most of them are small and operate underground even though there are about 10 declared brothels in Madras, each having seven to eight girls. These are operated by influential people, and with the knowledge of the police. A large number of such girls come on a contract basis through brokers, mainly from Andhra Pradesh. Girls are also taken from Madras to other cities like Bombay where they are in great demand.

(c) Street girls operate in the open and cater largely to the lower socio-economic class. Such girls, numbering seven to eight hundred, mostly hang around bus stops or other regular pick-up points. A street girl will charge about 300 rupees a night, and sometimes even more, going upto Rs 500. It often happens that three or four clients get together and share the girl—the cost; and also the risk of HIV infection, both for the sex worker and her clients. In this respect, prostitution in Tamil Nadu is quite unlike in the northern states which have specified red light districts, with more girls and costing less. This probably reflects a generally less tolerant social attitude towards the sex trade in southern India. As a CAN official puts it, "Greater the stigma, more the customer has to pay."

Transvestites and eunuchs (i.e. transvestites who have undergone castration) form another category of sex workers in Madras. Called *Alis,* they are found in other parts of India as well. Madras has a large community of about 250 *Alis* mostly concentrated in Satya Nagar, close to the beach where they have commercial sex (mostly oral sex and masturbation). Almost all *Alis* become transvestites at an early age through the temple system described earlier for Maharashtra. Most *Alis* undergo castration, using traditional methods without any anaesthesia. Lately, however, modern medical facilities are also used.

Once a person becomes an *Ali,* she is stigmatized by society including her immediate family. Says a CAN official, "Police repression and abuse of *Alis is* higher in Madras, and compared to their counterparts in north India they are more stigmatised. They are subjected to more police repression and abuse by rowdies than other types of sex workers. Police identify *Alis* with AIDS; as a result, most of them have left the inner city and gone to nearby areas such as Nungambakkam (CAN is located here) where they are relatively safe.

The taboos of which they are a victim emanate mainly from middle class values, influenced by westernisation. For which reason *Alis* are more at peace in low income settlements. As most of them undergo castration, their urinary passage gets blocked from time to time, thus often requiring minor surgery. But they are not treated properly in the hospitals nor given treatment at urology clinics. As a result they often end up trying to treat themselves.

Probably due to social ostracism and general ill-treatment meted out to them, *Alis* have a closely knit social organisation among themselves. A CAN official says, "They have leaders called *gurus* who command a certain obedience from the community. Outreach work is easy to acheive through the intervention of *gurus* who derive their seniority on basis of the length of time for which they have been castrated. There are about five or six such *gurus* in a given area. *Alis* have also developed a language of their own which is not understood by others.

A social worker at CAN who is in charge of the *"Ali* component" of the programme adds, "Most *Alis* are in the 20 to 40 age group though some are much older. They happen to be very good entertainers, cooks and actors. Having always wanted to be females from a very early age, they often engage in feminine work with their mothers, like helping in the kitchen and other household work. Bashful whenever touched or encountered by men, they yearn to be females, and behave so.

Ending up as sex workers is a result of their deep isolation and inability to get regular employment. They also have this desire to adopt a daughter or daughter-in-law and have kinship with others in their society *(Jamad). As* a result one of them will always act as a mother or an aunt to one or the other Ali. Mostly illiterate, they marry men, acting as their "wives". Given their psychological makeup Alis enjoy a certain degree of rapport only with other females."

Males who have sex with males (MSMs, in CAN parlance)

According to CAN estimates the number of men who have sex with men in Madras could well exceed 3000. This includes both; men who have sex for commercial purposes, and those who have it just for pleasure. Explains the CAN director, "There is no homosexual or gay culture in India like in the West. But here in India it is more a way of doing rather than a way of thinking. One reason is that a wide gap exists between men and women, as a result of which men are often uncomfortable with women, socially or sexually. The other reason is that opportunities for having sex with women is rather limited. Another important reason is that sex with female sex workers is very expensive."

In the course of two ethnographic surveys conducted, CAN was able to identify 70 different pick-up points and locales for sex activity involving MSMs, including bars, restaurants, beaches, cinema halls, river banks, parks, and train compartments (usually luggage van). They were also able to identify several native categories: *panthis* (butch or those who are *manly),danga (fairy* or those who are effeminate and play the female role in sex). Then there are the "double deckers"(men who play both masculine and feminine roles *orardhanari* in Tamil). CAN has identified 10 major cruising areas for carrying out its work among MSMs. About 730 customers come daily to one such place by the beach, 300 more come to another park.

According to a CAN staff member working with MSMs: "Most of the customers are not interested in women; more so as they also do not have to spend much—only about 50 rupees—for a boy. And female prostitutes, unlike a boy, do not indulge in oral sex. Customers, who are often married, have sex in the park or on the beach. After six in the evening, other customers including teenagers, also arrive. Rich *dangas* often pay Rs three to four hundred to have sex with a man. In a cinema hall, such boys often put out their hand and touch the thighs of the man sitting next to them. And, if the latter is agreeable, the two go to the cinema toilet where the boy provides oral sex to the man."

Malaysia

According to government figures, the cumulative total of HIV cases as of 1994 was 6370 persons. Of these 5011 contracted the virus through IV drug use, 223 through sexual intercourse, 12 through organ transplants and blood transfusions, and 11 from mother-to-child. The country has 90 full-blown cases of AIDS. NGOs, however, believe that the numbers should be more since testing is usually limited to a captive audience of drug addicts, prisoners and sex workers. They estimate the actual figure to be around 9000. Furthermore, under-reporting, they say, could be due to the fact that insurance companies in Malaysia do not pay for AIDS-related deaths, making doctors reluctant to report HIV cases .

Prostitution

A reason for believing the NGOs is the scale of prostitution in the country. Although no region wise estimates are available, projections by a team of researchers from the University of Penang estimate it to be anywhere between 43,000 and 142,000. The number includes sex workers from all major ethnic groups in the country. Of the girls arrested in 1994, 192 were foreigners including Indonesians, Filipinos, Chinese, and Thais (nearly 50 per cent are Thai); another 142 were underaged girls. According to a social worker from TENAGANITA, the number of gigolos in Kuala Lumpur has also increased in recent years although no estimated are available.

NGOs consider prostitution to be of two types, organised and unorganised. The latter includes sex workers who rent rooms in 'rooming' houses or work as singers, dancers or waitresses in the karoke music lounges, etc. Organized prostitution, on the other hand, is a part of crime syndicates, with girls completely under their control.

Unorganized Prostitution

This type of prostitution is closely linked to Malaysia's rapid economic growth and urban development, a result of the expanding service and entertainment sectors. In 1992, for example, Kuala Lumpur had 364 bars, 80 coffee houses, 2387 restaurants, 194 video arcades, 93 discos or dance halls, 1320 hair dressing saloons and 60 massage parlours. Such places are regular cruising areas or pick-up points where clients could find a girl, sometimes through pimps.

The social status of the "front" determines the price to be paid. For example, bar prostitutes earn 700 to 1000 RM a month compared to 300 RM earned by a street walker. Practically all important towns in the country including Johore, Penang and Ipoh are known to be centers of commercial sex.

Kuala Lumpur also has two red light areas, Chowkit and Petaling Jaya. Chowkit is situated in the older section of the town where Chinese Malays predominate. There are long rows of rooming houses *(rumah)* which are actually fronts for brothels. In 1992, there were 230 such houses'registered with Kuala Lumpur's municipality. Each such establishment has between five to ten girls, many of who rent the room only for the day. About 1000 transsexuals (all males) and 500 female sex workers operate in Chowkit.

Migrant workers, mainly from the Philippines~ also engage in prostitution during their free time. They are mostly younger than the full-time sex workers, and are taken to the brothels by pimps who hang around work places. In two or three days they earn as much as what they would have done in a whole month at a factory. They do not work as full-time sex workers because the papers mention their coming to the country for working in a factory. TENAGANITA's social worker adds, "They come here for three years or so, after which they return to their native country. Every year they are tested for HIV, and there are cases of maids from other countries who test positive".

Organised Prostitution

Organised prostitution takes place in high class hotels, apartment buildings and car parks. This involves a network of pimps, brokers and hotel and apartment complex managers who are in touch with one another through bell boys and walkie talkies. They take a commission from the girls who are kept as prisoners and have been forced into the profession. These girls are mostly from rural areas and totally ignorant of the city. They are taken around from one hotel to another in the night and have no idea of their whereabouts. Coming on the promise of a job, they are cheated into prostitution and are put into a brothel instead.

With nowhere to go, some of them have been trafficked overseas to Japan and the Middle East. During the last five years 3000 girls have been reported missing from Malaysia. Every year about 500 girls are 'lost'. TENAGANITA had intervened on behalf of one such group of Filipinos and helped them return to their own country. Usually, employment agencies recruit girls saying they do not have to pay any fees and will get work as a hotel receptionist or something similar. On arrival, however, they are confined to rooms and warned that unless they service at least 85 clients, they will not be allowed to leave.

Working Conditions

Working conditions for sex workers in the unorganised sector are much better in terms of physical environment than the dismal, overcrowded rooms in the brothels of Bombay or Surat. The girls earn much more money. But they have other problems, chief among them-being the constant fear of police arrest. Women with condoms are automatically arrested and remanded. They are afraid of even coming in groups to TENAGANITA's drop-in center, and therefore come individually. Transsexual sex workers, however have less fear.

Sex workers work full-time, part-time, or during weekends. Girls may live in one hotel and operate from another. Some live in the brothel itself while others come in only for sex work. The daily rent for a room is 25 dollars. And for each customer, the brothel owner or operator charges five dollars from the girl. He is also the time keeper, knocking at the door after 45 minutes have passed.

According to the NGO's field worker cum counsellor, "Self esteem among female sex workers is low." Is this due to their awareness about HIV? Low self-esteem may be due to a history of rape, having run away from home, or being pushed into the trade. Many of them have been raped by boyfriends and discarded. Women drug users often get into prostitution to sustain the habit or, when their husbands are taken into police custody, to support themselves and the children. TENANGITA tried job placement for some sex workers but failed since society generally refuses to accept them.

The whole psychology of sex workers is different and the dynamics difficult to understand. There is something about them which wants to return to all the violence and wretched life. Those who go into rehabilitation centers also want to come back. The life of the city-based female sex worker is a lonely one even though many of them share their earnings with others. A worker recalls how one girl, who was later found to be HIV positive, had to be picked up by an NGO personnel as she lay on the road. She had no friends to speak of. Sex workers need to be reconciled with their families, especially when found to be HIV positive. This is one area which, TENANGITA feels, needs to be addressed.

Speaking of violence and negativity, the counsellor states: "Clients beat them up if they insist on condom use. One fellow broke a girl's nose, and yet the hotel owner would not come to her rescue. A second woman had her teeth knocked off by a customer. There were two cases where sex workers were taken to a park and gang raped. The police did not take any action saying 'How can a sex worker be raped?' Women are mostly in a poor bargaining position and, even in poor health condition, the men insist on having them. Pregnant women particularly are in much demand. One such woman gave birth to a child just after a customer left her.

The women have little or no regard for themselves, just as one of them said to the counsellor,"If you can put my mind, body and spirit together, that will be the day". Another said, "My body and soul are separate". With their bodies so much abused another asked, "Can you restore my dignity? Maybe it will happen not in this life but in the next one." They have mostly been abused from a very young age. Women hooked on drugs, and engaged in sex work are detached from their bodies. Some bring their children along and drug the child till they finish work. These children stay in the room or run around in the street; some grow up to become prostitutes or pimps.

Continuing in the same vein, the counsellor said, "In addition to assaults from clients, sex workers also undergo harassment by police and brothel owners. Clients are spared while sex workers are arrested even when servicing the former in the brothel. The man is allowed to dress quietly while the girl has to grab a towel. Next morning the magistrate looks at the partly dressed female and orders 'Just get her out' ! Last year, a transsexual was arrested by the police, locked up and raped several times by a police officer and an immigration officer. She was a migrant from Indonesia".

Transsexuals and MSMs

According to a PINK TRIANGLE (PT) source, the transsexual community in Kuala Lumpur mainly comprises people who have migrated from different states in Malaysia. These people leave their own village or community because of the social stigma attached to being a transsexual. Some of them become sex workers because society is intolerant of their attitudes and fights shy of hiring them. Many indulge in commercial sex to earn enough money so that they can go to Singapore and get operated. They live in rooms with several of their own group, and it is here that clients come to them for sex. Earlier, they did the soliciting on the streets but that exposed them to police arrests, and rape and assault by clients who often came in a group and took them in a taxi to some remote place. Many transsexuals are also drug users.

There are some gay bars in Kuala Lumpur where MSMs come and find clients. Their exact number is not known, but it is relatively small. Sex takes place in hotel rooms, parking lots or in the homes of clients. The activity is completely underground, homosexuality being a crime according to Muslim law prevailing in Malaysia.

Thailand

Thailand is expected to have two million cases of HIV by the year 2000. According to Greg Carl (G.C), who works as a counsellor at the Thai Red Cross Society in Bangkok, serosurveillance of military conscripts, coming from all provinces and seen as representating the Thai male population, has shown HIV positivity rates between 1.5 and 2.0 per cent. Northern Thailand has the highest rate, followed by central, north east and lower Thailand. But, according to him, "Not enough people are being tested". Among women attending antenatal clinics, again the north accounts for the highest, and infection rates among pregnant women is similar to that of military conscripts. According to a survey by the Red Cross, as many as 70 per cent of Thai men were initiated into sex- through a sex worker. "After that first experience they have casual sex with girl friends" says Carl.

Estimates about the number of sex workers vary, with a 1991 study putting it at about 150,000. A subsequent study conducted by WHO puts the figure at an astounding 800,000, which is half of Thailand's female populationt According to Carl it could be no more than 200,000.

He sees prostitution as of two types, direct and indirect. In the former only sexual services are offered, and the customer chooses the sex partner. Indirect prostitution involves places which offer other services including massage parlours, coffee shops, and gogo bars. In such places, the customer has to negotiate with the sex worker and/or owner. The dividing line between the two, he feels, is very thin. Direct prostitution costs less because each girl has about 10 to 15 customers a night. Most of them are from the lower classes, and the rate for each girl varies from 60 to 80 bhat. In indirect prostitution, the charges range anywhere between 100 and 1000 bhat per girl for a night. Such girls never have more than two or three customers per night. These establishments are more flexible with the sex workers able to negotiate on how many days or nights they work, and are free to decide when they come or go. Such sex workers are more mobile and on the lookout for places where she or he can get better wages.

A slightly different perspective was provided by an official from EMPOWER: "Brothel girls live under more repressed control. They are paid about 20 bhat per customer, but never get to see the money; only counting the number of times they have serviced customers. And, they do not get the money unless they ask for it. It is a slave like condition; a system which gets protection from the police. In Chiang Mai, for instance, women working in tea houses are confined indoors with no freedom to go out. They have to work in very poor health conditions also, with only a small place for sleeping and servicing customers. When taken into custody after police raids, the time spent in confinement is considered to be a loss of work hours, which has to be made up for later. And if the owner happens to bail them out, then the girls are even more indebted to him. It is the same case when they go to see a doctor."

Working conditions for those in bars are equally oppressive although they have relatively more freedom. The official continues, "If a girl refuses to have sex with a customer, she loses money. The bar girls have to go with customers at least four times a month, failing which 300 or 400 bhat are deducted from the salary. If they happen to be late they are fined at the rate of two bhat per minute just as they are fined 50 bhat for eating late meals. If they are late at the dance floor, one bhat per song is deducted. At night they have to serve drinks to customers; at least 50 drinks per night, for which they get 50 bhat a month. And if she goes out with a customer all she gets is a commission." EMPOWER estimates that about half the girls in bars are married whereas in brothels a majority are not. Women in both categories support many relatives which often include in-laws. They do not tell their families about the work they do, but pretend to be working in a factory or restaurant.

Greig Carl also sees some major differences between male and female sex workers. "Male sex workers enter into prostitution mostly for economic reasons, wanting to help out their families. He may be the eldest child in the family with many mouths to feed. With drought and poor harvest, as happened in north-east Thailand two years ago, the family often moves to the big city. The boy, without skills or schooling, and no contacts either, cannot get any employment. Neither does the family have any savings to depend on for long. The boy, looking in the street for work meets people who suggest employment in a bar, where soon he gets picked up for sex. Some decide to stay on, hoping to return some day when they can start a business or get more education.

"However, studies show that they get addicted to a certain life style: getting attention, money and nice clothes to wear; going out to bars, movies, and restaurants. Coming, as they do, mostly from the poorest regions particularly in the north-east, a city like Bangkok has its own charms. They feel as if they have become a somebody, rather than remaining a nondescript farmer. It is hard to get back after that. The money they send home is much more compared to what they make from farming. The yearly income from farming is usually 2500 bhat; while now these families get between 2000 and 5000 bhat per month from the boys alone. This builds up family expectations; they want a new house, a TV; there is no end to it. Life becomes associated with consumer goods; they want a piece of Bangkok itself. And sex work is one way of getting money fast and easy. They, however, try to get away with as little sex work as possible and instead get as much money."

This is true of female sex workers as well, though many of them are sold or forced into prostitution. The consequences of being in bondage according to the ACCESS Director: "Some girls are bonded because their parents receive lump sum money from an agent in exchange of the girl. The family may be paid about 25,000 bhat, and the girl has to work till she earns twice that amount. Which means, even if she gets HIV she has to work till her debt is paid off. Half of her earnings go towards payment of the original debt while the other half goes into paying up the establishment cost of where she works.

"A girl likes to return home to her village v .. honour and dignity. Which means she has to go back after hav ; accumulated some wealth for the family. If she goes back without a..ything, people in the village will start whispering about her. In recent times, thanks to the AIDS scare, a girl coming back home sooner than expected is presumed to have HIV. If instead she has money, buys land, builds a house, and has cattle or buffalo, then she can go back with dignity. For girls who are bonded this takes several years, most of them not having enough funds to work independently. In northern Thailand they very often begin as sex workers bonded to an agent. That is when they are at highest risk, having to work at tea houses where customers mostly come from the lower classes."

According to Carl, most women go back home after 'retiring'. There are many communities which have sex workers returning home, keeping alive the belief that sex work is an easy source of income. On reaching 25 years of age most sex workers start getting fewer clients, even though some men prefer older women. Many hope to find a foreign client who will be their boyfriend and, some day, take them out of prostitution. If they return home before that, they get married and settle down.

Some actually enter into prostitution to make enough money to get an education. Education is free upto level six only, after which they have to pay; and it becomes rather expensive. There are also those who do sex work seasonally, for short periods. Since they are desperate for the money, they choose the peak tourist season. Thais also go out of the country and are recruited by brokers to work in Japah, Taiwan and even Malaysia. Sometimes they are cheated and forced to work as sex workers.

Contrasting the two sexes, Carl explains: "Male sex workers think of themselves as individuals and are on the lookout for that one customer who will be their saviour. It suits their lifestyle to be alone, to feel that they are in control of their lives, to be independent and work when they want to." But this again depends on the establishment they are working for. "In some places, the boys come and go whenever they feel like it. In others, if they miss three nights in a week, they are thrown out". Thai society is less accepting of male sex workers than their female counterparts. Says Carl, "The general image is that male sex workers are homosexuals or are effeminate (*gaturi*, the term for transvestite). But this is not absolutely true.

"Rural Thais cannot accept people being gay. *Gaturis* are considered to be second class women, but being gay is just outrageous. It is believed that the first-born son should get married, and therefore, a homosexual son is seen as a shame for the family. For which reason a lot of homosexuals or bisexuals get married. A majority of sex workers, however, are heterosexual or bisexual; others being *gaturi* or gay. A majority of male sex workers regard themselves as heterosexual; and have girlfriends, wives and even children. Although one Thai study claims that male sex workers become homosexuals, it is hard to believe so. While homosexual sex workers have emotional needs, a heterosexual one has a wife or a girlfriend. The latter considers sex as work; and Thais are good at separating work from emotion. Even women who are normally shy will go and dance at a gogo bar. And men, if you get them alone, break down, remorseful about their work."

Girls from northern Thailand are more favoured for sex work than those from other parts of the country. Carl attributes this to cultural and physical traits: "In terms of skin colour and personal habits, women from the north are highly desirable, for which reason they are brought to Bangkok"

In general, rural Thai society has special expectations from daughters. Women are seen as the basic providers, a fact which may be attributed to their dominant role in agriculture. According to a woman counsellor at the Red Cross Society: "In some rural areas the girl has to do a good turn to her parents, work for them. By sending money, even working as a prostitute, she shows gratitude to the parents. Even after giving up prostitution, a girl will visit her parents, and everybody sees her as a good girl". Society's expectations from women partly accounts for girls leaving school at an early age and starting as sex workers as early as the age of 12. She adds "We have to try and change the attitudes of parents and to make secondary education compulsory. We have to reduce the supply of prostitutes"

Srilanka

Located at the southern tip of the Indian subcontinent, this island nation has not been spared from the epidemic. Of a total population of 17 million, however, the reported number of HIV/ AIDS cases has been relatively low—155 persons, of whom 25 were foreign nationals. Judging by their backgrounds one may assume that the primary source of infection was foreign travel for the purpose of employment or business. About five of these reported HIV cases had been local sex workers.

The sex industry, though illegal, is spread throughout the country with high concentration in urban centres like the capital Colombo and the south-western coastal belt which thrives on tourism.

Tourism is also the third highest source of foreign exchange earning for the country. The exact number of sex workers in the country is not known, but rough estimates by researcher, Professor Ratnapala, places the figure around 20,000 (personal communication).

According to a study conducted by the author in 1987, "In five out of the total 47 municipal wards in Colombo, there are 68 brothels and over 100 hotels and guest houses where prostitution takes place. Police officials estimate that in the 68 brothels alone over 2000 girls are engaged in prostitution; many earning a regular monthly wage from the operators. Migrant prostitution is also common. The operators shunt girls back and forth from one location to another depending on the tourist season or local religious festivals. Some moonlighting by office girls is also done in the city. This is in contrast to older patterns of prostitution in Sri Lanka when the trade was limited to street walkers found along a few city roads after dark" (Weeramunda 1990:5).

From a reconnaissance survey done in January 1994 of the five coastal towns along the Southern Province, the total number of sex workers was placed at or around 600. Of this a large proportion (390) were males. However, with each additional month of intervention, this number tended to increase. Information was gathered about brothels where, it was found, between 10 and 15 girls worked; or about syndicates providing small groups of children to foreign clients. Thus, if one were to map out all the settings where prostitution takes place in both rural and urban Sri Lanka, 20,000 would be a conservative estimate.

The entry of males and children into the sex trade is a development closely associated with the upsurge of tourism in the late sixties. The trade also includes some effeminate males called *ponnayas,* who function like the *Alis* of Madras: providing oral, and sometimes anal sex to the local men. All forms of prostitution are covert in nature due to various factors including its being illegal, social condemnation and stigmatisation, etc. Also a result of frequent police crackdowns, especially on street walkers and women working in brothels.

With the advent of the "AIDS scare", crackdowns on child prostitution in the tourist belt have increased, some of these operations being spearheaded by local "task forces". However, this has only contributed to the flourishing of organised crime syndicates. Some establishments, for instance, operate with police protection and/or patronage of influential people.

Invariably, it is the unpriviledged, self-employed sex worker, usually female, who faces the brunt of the law and law enforcement authorities. A noteworthy feature when applying the law is the lack of severity in dealing with beach boys who are essentially male prostitutes.

Although different value orientations may apply to male and female sex workers, the factors which push them into prostitution are akin to those prevalent in other Asian societies. Poverty is a common background variable, and usually it is not absolute but relative poverty. The precipitating factors for most females are premature sexual encounters and loss of virginity, failed marriages and loss of support from kinsmen, and premature widowhood—particularly as a consequence of the continuing ethnic war in the North where as many as 20,000 men have lost their lives. A hidden network of brokers and pimps promotes the incorporation of such women into the industry either at brothels or as streetwalkers. In the case of "beach boys", the initiation begins at an early age—as early as 10 years—leading to early school leaving and taking on full-time sex work with foreign male and/or female clients. They are procured from the beaches or at small guest houses or hotels in the tourist belt.

Invariably, children and young adults who enter the industry are mostly from economically marginalised rural families living on the periphery of the tourist belt. According to a pilot study done in 1993 by the author, the average monthly earning of such families was about 60 US dollars. Earnings from prostitution, however, was much higher-with children earning an average of four US dollars per sexual act (see Weeramunda 1994). Beach boys may earn as much as 200 US dollars per month during the peak tourist season. Female sex workers earn about the same amount if they go with foreign clients, although earnings from local clients are much less.

IV. BUILDING TRUST AMONG SEX WORKERS

NGOs vary in their approach to building trust and winning the confidence of sex workers. It depends on the number and kind of personnel they have, the type of sex worker being dealt with, and the context (physical, social and political) in which inlterventions take place. In any event, trust is essential for launching any activity inviting participation of sex workers in planning and implementing such enterprises. The experience of each NGO in this regard will be discussed separately as follows.

IHO

IHO's contact with the sex workers of Bombay first started in the early eighties with a health education programme for them. The IHO director recalls "According to the information gathered at the camp, we found that a number of girls had been forced into prostitution. Others had come through the religious system of exploitation; and a number of them were minors. Some had a history of rape, failed marriages or abduction. There is international trafficking through which girls are brought from Bangladesh and Nepal, and sold here in Bombay; others have been sent to the Middle-East countries. We soon realized that unless we worked on sex and police harassment issues, we could not work on medical and health aspects."

A concrete plan of action was adopted by IHO by venturing directly into the field. They first went to the Belgaum District in Karnataka where on a particular day between 3000 and 5000 girls are dedicated to the Goddess *Yellamma (Kali)*. After this they went to Nepal to find out why and how girls were being sent to India. Social action then followed, and some minors in prostitution were sent back to their families, and some girls were sent back to Nepal.

Work with a designated population of sex workers began only in the late eighties. Till 1989 a hit-and-run approach was followed since there was no staff, clinic or transport. They had only two camps a year. In l990, they started a condom promotion programme when AIDS became a serious problem in India. In 1991, the *Saheli* Project was started.

When IHO's field staff first entered the red light areas of Bombay the community regarded them with distrust. Recalls one doctor, "They used to think we were police people. They were an exploited group so why should they trust outsiders?" A perspective on the first interactions was provided by a sex worker who is now a peer educator "When IHO workers first came here, I did not believe they were going to do any good. I also rejected them saying 'I don't want anything from you'. But they did not give up coming here and slowly became friendly. They called me sister or mother and built a relationship. I had not heard these words from society. People only come for sex. This was new."

Working through a kinship terminology was particularly helpful since most sex workers would have lost or given up contact with their own families and relatives, a vacuum which the IHO staff was able to fill. The staff took one further step by ritually bonding the relationship through the *raksha bandhan* ceremony. The ritual takes place in Hindu households on the first full moon day after the rainy season when fishermen go out to sea for the first time. The sister comes with a lighted lamp and waves it around the brother in reverence and gives him sweets to eat. She then touches his feet and he gives her his blessing and assurance of protection throughout her life. As one IHO member put it: "We went to them as brothers seeking their welfare and health."

In this context how did IHO's female staff fit in? Recalled one of them, "Initially, they were afraid of us, not wanting to hear of condoms or AIDS. But gradually we mingled with them; giving them affection, touching them, loving them like a sister, and asked them general questions about their life, their health, so that they became close. Many of the girls were depressed not having got any love or affection from society. The person who brought them being a man, they were suspicious of men. We talked to them hoping to change that attitude. We took the girl's side".

Social ties ritually consolidated in this manner was a first step to building trust in a culturally accepted and meaningful way. The delivery of other services such as STD treatment, condoms, counselling, sero testing, and handling personal problems relating to work and lives of sex workers were thus placed within a larger framework of care and protection just as between siblings.

Another step was involving brothel managers in implementing the safe sex programme. IHO identified leaders from three different levels: sex workers, brothel managers, and brothel owners. Placing several people at one level in the charge of a leader from the next higher level, but using the same ideology of care and protection (those in charge of *sahelis* were called *tai* meaning "elder sister") rather than the existing framework of exploitation. In this manner, IHO was able to win the cooperation of brothel managers for the safe sex programme.

If they had been ignored the outcomes would perhaps not have been as effective.

GAP

GAP's experience in building trust among sex workers has been limited to one year, during which time a social worker concentrated on the red light areas of Surat. Initial contact with the community was made through a social worker from another NGO who had worked there earlier, rehabilitating sex workers at remand homes. Through this person, GAP met the brothel managers in Surat. Recalling the first meeting, GAP's director said, "We made them learn about the disease and asked them what they thought of it. The proposals then came from them. We asked 'Do you need us nor not? Are your children getting proper education? Do you want them to get a proper education? If you are suffering from a disease, do you want to go to a hospital? Do you have a school here? Do your children attend that school' ?"

When health authorities began to subject sex workers to blood tests GAP intervened, since it did not accept testing in principle. Later, the interruption was less confrontational and more on a person-to-person basis. The social worker focussed on building personal relationships with a few girls in one small brothel. She would visit them every day in the morning hours when they were relatively free, sit and chat about their daily problems like getting a baby or dealing with some sickness. She took toys and English books for the children. In about six months she was able to talk about their personal health problems. She met one girl who complained of an illness, which she thought could be STD, but which others in the brothel thought was AIDS. She took the girl personally to the government STD clinic in the city and had her examined and treated.

Visiting the brothel area with the social worker, she saw the effectiveness of the help given. Quoting from her field notes: It is about 6.30 in the evening. Some women are standing on the porches dressed and waiting for customers. I approach one of the brothels through a back alley in the company of S, the social worker. Suddenly, a young female in her early twenties, leaves her small group of friends, rushes out and hugs S warmly and keeps holding her hands and talking excitedly. Another girl joins and invites us inside. On the way up the steps to the brothel, S trips and hits her leg against an iron railing. Both girls hold S and ask whether she is alright. One girl, whom S had earlier helped to conceive and deliver a baby, strokes her (S's) legs and hands. While a customer waits inside talking to another girl, one of the girls asks him to leave remarking, "They come here for sex. You come here as our friend!" This is only the beginning of the long road to gaining acceptance and friendship among the community of sex workers in Surat.

CAN

According to CAN, strategies for gaining trust vary, depending on the type of sex worker. Female sex workers cannot be approached directly due to the fact that they operate secretly. Contacts had to be first established with the brokers and owners of hotels which were used for sex. While doing an ethnography, male social workers from CAN posed as clients to establish friendly relations with brokers and hotel owners. Contacting family girls (who posed as members of a family), was done through *aunties* or female brokers. Said one social worker "Getting the first contact with family girls was difficult. Once trust was built with *aunties,* it was easy. Every family girl knows at least 10 other similar girls".

ContactingAlis was initially done by male social workers, but it later turned out that *Alis* were much more trusting of female social workers rather than males. Contact with *Alis* was also easy by working through the *gurus*, their leaders. Building trust with MSMs was done by employing educated males, who were also MSMs, as social workers. They knew the networks and circuits, and helped CAN to identify peer educators for the programme. In addition, CAN built up close friendly links with people in the vicinity of the scene of prostitution; such as shopkeepers, bar and hotel owners, and security guards in parks and beach areas.

SIAAP

Approaching sex workers who operate underground was no easy task for M, SIAPP's social worker who recounted her travails thus: "We started work two years ago, and not knowing where to begin, I went to Parry's Corner, a cruising area for street girls. I went in the evenings, all alone, and just observed things for several days. I introduced myself to the girls and said.'We want to help you'. Some girls said, OK and asked what they could do. I said 'I would like to know more about you'. From then on, everyday I just went and talked to them, taking care not to jot down any notes. Some of them even took me to a restaurant nearby and offered tea.

A few days later, I took along a packet of *nirodh* (condoms) and *bindi* (coloured dot worn on the forehead by Asian women) and gave it to them". Later, talking about AIDS, she explained that condoms were the only protection against it. But they professed to be using it already.

Asked if she could bring the packets everyday, they said "Yes", and by and by they just came around to talk to her. Once, just after she left, the police raided the girls making them suspicious of her. After this they didn't come near her for some time. She remembers "While I waited for them, they would see men trying to solicit me, pull me by the hand and harass me". Seeing this the girls understood her true position. Realizing that the best thing to do was to recruit some intelligent and friendly girls as peer educators, she got two volunteers and trained them. "At the end of three months we had contacted 150 women."

However, according to the SIAAP director, recent experiences in new areas, particularly in the four southern states, has been remarkably and consistently different, leading to a change in strategy. Presently, at least among sex workers in the southern states, there is a remarkable climate of acceptance, faith and trust. And the response of the women to interactions in the short term, and later in the long term has been very positive and encouraging. This, she feels, is the single largest factor responsible for building trust. She says, "The truth really is that the community's trust in us usually exceeds our own (NGOs and others outside)."

According to her the women were approached directly after a process of revealing credentials. They were then told the purpose and asked if they would be interested in woking together for their own protection as well as that of others in the community. Nearly all women responded positively and accepted the condoms. They understood the risks involved and actively helped in contacting other women as well and educating and providing them with condoms.

The building of trust has come through:

(a) Transparency of intent.
(b) No hidden agendas like moral reform, rehabilitation, etc.
(c) Consistent and persistent outreach.
(d) Distribution of good quality *Nirodh* (condom).

(e) Providing a safe space where women can get together.
(f) Discussing empowerment through collectivisation and helping the process further.
(g) Providing authentic treatments for STDs.
(h) Raising self esteem by giving the women space, time and support to undergo a process of deconstruction and reconstruction of identity.
(i) Continuous liaison with the policy to minimise the violence on women.
(j) Equipping women with new social skills and the ability to work effectively in the area of STDs/HIV impact minimisation.

These are some of the strategies more significantly critical than sentiments alone.

Tenaganita

Working alone, and when she had free time, TENAGANITA's counsellor cum social worker began to establish contact with sex workers in the Chowkit red light area. That was two years ago. She recalled her strategy: "You have to go through some friend of the sex workers. I used to just sit at a tea stall and wait, and once they got to know me they came and talked. They need someone to talk to. About 150 sex workers were thus contacted in the course of two years".

Pink Triangle (PT)

Initial contact with transsexuals and female sex workers took place about two years ago. Gaining the trust of the former was relatively easy, but the latter had to be approached through the prostitution network including brothel owners and pimps. One of PT's social worker remembers "First we had to be friends with them; otherwise they do not trust you. There was resistance in the beginning. They could not understand why we should be there in the first place." But then the safe sex programme was explained individually to 50 brothels owners in a persuasive non-confrontational manner. That is how their cooperation was obtained to distribute condoms among female sex workers working in their establishments. Pimps were similarly educated about the programme.

Recalling her experiences, a social worker said, "The girls were agreeable and responded even better if I talked to them about their children and the needs of dependents at home". Another social worker, a transsexual, who had been a sex worker, had contacts with both transsexual and female sex workers. According to her, during the initial stages an assessment was made about the needs of the specific population. This included: what they knew about AIDS, problems about condom use, use of lubricants, why they were reluctant to use or carry condoms, or if they were too poor to buy them, or did they douche after sex and with what? These discussions were then used to draw up a questionnaire. Involving sex workers in fact-finding and implementation was a novel way of gaining their trust.

Thai Red Cross Society

In the course of a sentinel surveillance in 1993, G.C, one of the NGOs social workers, started a pilot activity in two gay bars of Bangkok.-The assignment included talking on STD, AIDS, condom use, and giving condom demonstration for patrons. He recalls, "We got to know the managers who invited us to talk to the boys (male sex workers) and to promote ideas on safe sex among them. I went as a foreigner and as a customer. Speaking Thai and as a gay I made attempts to recruit peer educators; the captain of a bar who was my main contact, and at another bar a sex worker. I got condom kits from abroad; and tried to promote skills such as making herbal shampoo to impress on the boys the idea of a good life.

"In one bar, the manager was cooperative but did not want to take responsibility for the programme. In the second one, the results were more disheartening. The only contact, a sex worker, had left the bar and the manager blamed me for it. I was not allowed to talk to the boys or distribute condoms after that. The manager also had sex with the boys (like a test run) and he did not want to use condoms. He had started as a singer, then a sex worker, and was finally running his own bar."

Going through the management is an important step in gaining access to such establishments; which also feel threatened by the presence of change agents. At the same time managements want to take little responsibility in intervention efforts, which means that the total burden falls on the change agent's shoulders. The fact that the change agent in this instance went as a gay client also helped in gaining trust.

Empower

The NGO deals with sex workers in bars and brothels and not with street girls who are not easily accessible. In order to fulfill its outreach activities among the girls in bars and brothels, the staff had to win the cooperation rnd trust of the owners and managers (many owners are non-Thai while managers are usually Thai). As the Coordinator put it: 'We had to negotiate with owners and managers before gaining access. They were suspicious, and had to be convinced that we were working to protect the women from disease rather than attacking the owners. Needing the support of owners and customers, we informed them that the objective was giving the sex workers a better living and better business. The hardest thing is getting around owners to change their business attitude whereby they do not (excessively) profit out of the women. While the sex industry continues to expand it is mainly the owners who have money and influence".

Once trust and friendship was established, the staff was allowed to visit the women. Space was also provided by the owners in Pat Pong area to set up a small office. The idea was to create close contact with the sex workers, allow easy access to the center; and become part of the community—know what their real problems were. The Coordinator continued, "We were outsiders who knew things only from the perspective of our own kind of people. It was only when we became a part of their community did we realize that they could not do simple things like having an account in a bank or filling a form at a post office." EMPOWER's activities were thus guided by the basic needs of sex workers and finding ways to fulfil them.

Access

The NGO began safe sex interventions in Phayao, a town in Chiang Kom district of northern Thailand. Phayao has about 20 brothels situated close to one another with about five or six girls working in each of them. The sex workers were contacted through a brothel owner's association which had been formed earlier by a local public health officer. The owners were already aware of the need to take preventive action against HIV. The NGO had a team of ex-sex workers (female) who visited the brothel girls in the afternoon, talked to them, and provided them with condoms.

However, when the team moved to another town in Pan district (Chiang gai) they faced a lot of hostility from brothel owners. The essential ingredients for cooperation were missing here: no formal organization among owners and a lack of awareness about HIV. The mood had been aggravated by a BBC programme which had been filmed at the brothels without their knowledge. The team had to therefore abandon its work there. Small as it is, this example highlights the strategies which are relevant in brothel type situations and that it is not impossible to get the cooperation of managers once they are educated about HIV.

CFPA

Given the secretive nature of the sex trade in Sri Lanka, CFPA's methods of gaining the trust of sex workers was similar to those of the South Indian NGOs. Knowledge about the social groups and settings in which prostitution took place was painstakingly gathered by a team of four field coordinators and eight counsellors through informal talks with minor government officials and grass root health personnel such as midwives, and through informal community leaders. During the first three months of fieldwork, several small groups and communities were identified for intervention within the Southern Province.

Small groups of beach boys numbering 25 to 50 were located near the resort towns of Bentota, Hikkaduwa, Polhena, and Batigama. Another location was a low income community of about 100 households near the town of Dondra (about 20 kms south of Galle), a few of which depended on prostitution for their livelihood. Customers would either come for sex to the homes or they would take the women out to another place. Another point of intervention was the STD clinic at the government hospital in Karapitiya near Galle town. Since some of the patients were sex workers, it was assumed that entry into their social domain would be made possible by talking to them at the clinic.

But several obstacles had to be overcome before the change agent could gain the trust of sex workers. Chief among these was the fear that intervention would pose a threat to their livelihood or security. The counsellors had to visit the groups or communities frequently, socialize with them, accept food or drinks offered, listen and empathize. In short, be willing to see things from the sex workers' perspective. Talking about STDs and AIDS was avoided to a great extent, and instead other issues of relevance to the sex workers were discussed. These included problems with law enforcement, housing, children's education, and domestic or family conflicts. The counsellors shared such problems with the sex workers and, wherever possible, assisted them in finding solutions (for example, finding a school for a child who had dropped out for several years). In fact, initial attempts to discuss AIDS or STDs drew negative responses from the sex workers who either said "We know everything about it; so there is no point talking" or "Some doctors came and tested our blood and did not find AIDS. So what we do cannot possibly lead to us get it."

Counsellors themselves were an obstacle in gaining the trust of sex workers. Most of them came from middle class back grounds, with school education and a "respectable job". As a consequence, they had difficulty in relating to groups they were conditioned to stigmatize or would not have otherwise socialised with. Contacting sex workers on the beat was well nigh impossible for almost all of them; relating to them on a one-to-one basis as equals was even more difficult. Instead, they felt more comfortable in the role of "educator" or "counsellor" which had an element of social superiority inbuilt.

A third obstacle was the community attitude towards sex workers. For them subjecting sex workers to blood tests was an acceptable strategy for HIV prevention. Any type of socializing with them was, on the other hand, out of form. This was clearly demonstrated by the fact that CFPA had to shift its outreach center at Hikkaduwa on two occasions within a year due to opposition from landlords and neighbours when sex workers began dropping in for chats or came to attend workshops. Changing public attitudes to prostitution was certainly not within the scope of the intervention programme.

Mere socializing and establishing friendship with sex workers was only an emotive element essential to gain trust. Real trust began only when the sex workers were accepted as team members and given a role in implementing the programmes. This was made possible by adopting the peer educator model, a result of the author's familiarisation tour in other Asian contexts described later. That an external agency was willing to recognize their leadership potential; gaining knowledge and teaching others, was a new challenge. They had always been ostracized, bullied and made to think of themselves as criminals. The exercise proved that trust can only be established when two parties work as equals in a spirit of sharing and learning from each other.

V. NGO SUPPORT FOR SELF HELP INITIATIVE OF SEX WORKERS

In the South Asian context at least, sex workers are not initiative-oriented. This is perhaps due to the marginal status they hold in Asian societies. Initiatives were thus generated by the concerned NGOs as a consequence of their AIDS prevention activities. Although it is a moot question as to what extent such externally induced initiatives have been sustainable, self help moves have taken place in many important directions. These include promotion of condom use, fostering avenues for selfexpression, providing child care and health facilities, legal protection, education, self-employment, and promoting unionization.

IHO

In order to provide Bombay's sex workers with easy access to condoms, IHO started "Project *Saheli" (Saheli* meaning "Friend") in 1991. The strategy, in the words of one of its social workers, was "If one girl understands what is HIV or STDs she can pass on this knowledge to others. We realized that we had many girls under us. To supervise these girls or *sahelis,* we appointed *tais* (elder sisters) who belong to the middle rung as brothel managers and know much more about HIV or STDs than *sahelis.* The *tais* in turn help the *sahelis.* All *tais* are not sex workers and have to take on more responsibilities. They not only distribute condoms but also explain all about HIV to the *sahelis,* show them the STD albums provided, and insist that they promote condom use among sex workers."

IHO holds regular workshops for its. volunteer outreach workers, and involves them in the task of bringing condoms once a week by the mobile unit to the brothels. *sahelis* and *tais* counsel sex workers on their health problems and, if necessary, refer them for treatment at the STD clinic run by IHO at the local Salvation Army building. They also perform the opening ceremonies for workshops. Adds Dr. N., an IHO member: "If we have a function in our programme, we do not invite this or that minister. A minister will come for the occasion after which it is all out of his mind. Instead, we held a conference only for *sahelis* at the Max Mueller Building, presided over by a *saheli* as lectures were given by other *sahelis.* Every two weeks, the IHO social workers hold group meetings with the outreach workers in the brothels so that they can be in touch with the problems faced by them in the field context itself.

The aim has thus been to develop self awareness and self respect, which the IHO believes are prerequisites for self protection. Self awareness, has been further promoted through avenues for self expression. Not only by talking at workshops and seminars but also through the printed medium. The editor of IHO's newsletter comments: "We usually consider sex workers as irresponsible people who are the carriers and spread disease. This is not true. We thought of starting a magazine for them through which, we could know their real lives. They themselves provided the name for the magazine *Saki Saheli* which means friend or female companion. "Sex worker" sounds demeaning, not showing them any respect. The magazine is in two languages, Hindi and Marathi. When we came up with the first issue, we asked them to write their story, how they came into the business, and what they felt about being (HIV) positive.

One girl, who was positive wrote: "There are many dangers in life. AIDS is one more of those dangers". Another positive girl wrote: "This is our fate. We will live somehow." She wrote about how she came into the sex business; how the social workers got her tested, and finally the revelation that she was positive. At first it was a shock; but then, seeing other girls who were also positive she slowly accepted it. She wrote: "It was not my fault. There is no way out. It is not *karma;* it just happened." This way, other girls who are also positive and read about such suffering learn to live and cope with HIV better.

One obstacle to self expression is the language barrier. This is so because many girls do not speak Hindi or Marathi as they come from other states while some are from Nepal. Lack of literacy is also a handicap if the girl enters the sex trade very early in life, and particularly if she comes through the temple system. The editor recalled how such problems were overcome: "Our social workers would talk to them and write their stories. In the weekly meetings, the social workers read out the articles that had been written and edited them before the magazine was printed. I also read out the articles to get their reaction, whether a particular article should be included or not. The girls also write poems, or songs from films, often adding their own line about condoms or AIDS."

This type of participation has had a salutary effect on the sex workers who have elected to work as peer educators. Recalled one 33 year old, working as a *tai: "I* wanted to learn something and teach something, to do some good. I did not go to school, and only survived using my brains. With IHO I gained knowledge and new ideas. Before that I was illiterate and afraid of speaking. Now I can face anyone; earlier, I was living in a cage. If someone came to me asking something, I was afraid to reply. I don't care about that now".

A slightly older woman working as a *saheli* in another brothel recalled, "Because of IHO, we now get to go out. Before that, we did not go out or know about life outside the brothel. We just sat here all day long only cooking food and sometimes going to a temple. Now we know how to speak and how to make others aware. Much earlier, I had a desire to be a teacher or a leader. Now, even if the IHO does not give us condoms, we will buy and use them."

GAP

GAP's efforts at promoting self help initiatives are still in a formative stage and are limited to helping sex workers visit clinics for STD checks and treatment and helping individual children to gain literacy. They plan an open-air school for the children of sex workers in Surat's red light area, and operate a mobile service for STD treatment, medical help and immunization programmes for children. A mobile service is considered essential since the women do not move out of their surroundings unless they decide to go to another city. Condoms are distributed among sex workers free of charge by the Surat Municipality. To realize its objectives GAP needs money. The director estimates that additional work will mean an increase of its present budget of 400,000 rupees by nearly twice the amount.

CAN

For condom promotion, CAN has launched a unique strategy of selling condoms to female sex workers through brokers and other contacts in the prostitution networks, once the target population has been educated about the advantages of safe sex. However, among other types of sex workers such *as Alis* and MSMs, condoms are distributed free of charge. The rationale behind this difference in strategy is that customers who pay as much as 300 rupees for sex with a girl will not be unwilling to pay five or 10 rupees for a condom. CAN director elaborated, "If a person buys a condom, chances of his using them are high. Condoms are sold by brokers and sex workers; the customer has to pass these points. We do not determine how much the condom should be sold for, but usually it is between two and 10 rupees."

In the face of constant harassment of *Alis* by the Madras police, CAN has decided to take up their cause and has a lawyer assigned to defend them. One staff member stated: "If *Alis* are arrested while in the act of sex we cannot do anything. But the important thing is that they fight for themselves. They plan to form a union and have it registered very soon". CAN has also arranged with the Director of Madras STD control programme to treat *Alis* since many of them have STD but do not go to the clinic on their own for fear of rejection. If there are no medicines available at the hospital, CAN arranges for it free of cost. Adds the social worker in charge: "We want them to get good treatment; for which reason we personally take them to the clinic". CAN also hopes to hire the services of a beautician at the main office "since *Alis* do not like going out to a beautician on their own, afraid of being insulted." *Alis* will pay a nominal fee for this service. CAN has also started a savings scheme for sex workers.

Illiteracy and a negative social attitude have largely prevented *Alis* from getting employment. CAN expects to conduct a literacy programme for them and is coordinating with a number of companies to train them for jobs. CAN has also helpedAlis and MSMs to organize events which would give expression to their in-born talents as entertainers. Said the Director: "A function was organised exclusively for sex workers, bringing them to a common platform for creating awareness. Booking a theatre, a show was organized where the sex workers themselves produced a play. The story was about a king and queen whose son gets infected with AIDS. The hakim (doctor) is called who gives them information about AIDS.

"Other invitees to the play included brokers, pimps and brothel keepers. Once the message came in a traditional form, the people believed it. In between there were short film clips, slides and songs having AIDS messages and peer leaders saying: 'AIDS is our problem; it is going to affect us; and controlling it is in our hands.' As many as 400 sex workers organized it and they went around selling tickets to regular customers also. The Secretary of Health also came lending respectability to a people who are mostly treated like scum. We invited sex workers as people with dignity. CAN also organized a similar programme for people in the MSM circuit. It was a musical programme. The MSMs are good actors and entertainers who like to dance."

CAN has no immediate plans to initiate self help measures among other types of sex workers such as women and MSMs, although one official stated that at least 70 per cent of female sex workers would like to give up the job because of the attached social stigma.

CAN has also begun a support group for HIV positive MSMs. The group has non-positive people also to avoid stigmatization. Said one social worker: "We mix with them casually and even visit their homes. Their families, on seeing that, are convinced that no harm will come by having a positive person at home. Access to counselling in hospitals is limited. On being told you are positive the person becomes a mental wreck and even attempts suicide. The situation gets even worse when they are also thrown out of jobs." At present, the group consists of men only and meets every Sunday afternoon.

SIAAP

The principal aim of working among sex workers is the self-organisation of women. Currently major programmes in the cities of Tiruchirapalli, Madurai and Pondicherry are planned to be implemented entirely by sex workers. In these areas sex workers are well on the way to formalisation of collectives where sex workers themselves handle responsibilities and are paid wages at par with Programme Managers.

The first ever meeting of sex workers in Madras to discuss self-organisation was held on 15 August, 1994. Subsequently several such meetings were held in Madras, Pondicherry, Cuddalore, Coimbatore, Bangalore, Hyderabad and other programme areas. At these meetings self-organisation has been the central issue on the agenda with strategies to increase programme effectiveness being complementary.

At another level, women are increasingly seeking STD treatment at the Royapettah Government Hospital in Madras where SIAAP has a counselling centre. Interestingly most of these women are either referred to or brought by sex workers. An examination of the records at the hospital reveals a decline in the incidence of STDs among this group over a period of time. Sex workers here have used materials produced by the programme to negotiate with clients—lumpens, police and even lovers and husbands. They also educate other sex workers, who they may come across, about the advantages of condom use. Much of the initiation and supervision of the programmes is done together with sex workers who volunteer their time for the purpose.

Women have specifically recommended the supply of good quality condoms free of cost. It is not a management rationale that determines free supply versus social marketing of condoms. (In reality it is much easier to sell condoms than to purchase and later distribute them free of cost, particularly when they are not budgeted in the programme.)

Sex workers have invariably and unequivocally stated that free supply of good quality condoms and reduction of police harassment are two major factors that will improve the quality of their lives as individuals and lead to more effective treatment of STDs and HIV infections. As far as strategies go, sex workers are both the first to identify problems within a programme as well as to suggest solutions.

However, this can come about in a planned manner in which the sex worker is taken through the steps of identifying problems, discussing options and arriving at solutions. Most practical solutions to problems related with programmes come from the women themselves. Several such self-help initiatives are invaluable and critical to NGOs and form a major part of their work.

TENGANITA

The NGO is primarily concerned with the legal and human rights of sex workers in Malaysia who increasingly face police repression. In June, 1994, TENGANITA challenged the arrest of a sex worker. The director says, "Dealing with these concerns we had a legal session where lawyers came and told the sex workers of their rights. They even gave them a telephone line to call for help when arrested. We try to arrange legal representation for the sex workers. Some 21 (transsexual) sex workers were arrested one day and the lawyers.went at 8.00 in the morning to represent the 'girls'. Because the lawyers were there, the girls were produced at 12 noon; and the police changed the charge from soliciting to taking drugs.

"That meant an automatic remand for two weeks. The courts had urine tests done for drugs and only one of them was found to be positive. After a week, the rest were released. They (the sex workers) came back to us saying that this could not go on. Five of them decided to sue the police for unlawful arrest; since some of them were arrested from their own rooms while watching TV. We wanted to challenge the soliciting allegation, saying that the client should also be charged. The Bar Association was angry with us for supporting 'unwanted elements'. As a result, sex workers have been going underground, leading to more criminalisation and greater chances of organized prostitution, which means less and less access to women."

The population referred to were transsexuals who are more outgoing and conscious of their rights than female sex workers. They had their own association till recently to provide mutual assistance to members. The NGO has also provided condoms free of charge to both transsexual and female sex workers through its network of social workers and counsellors. Among the latter, condoms are promoted as a means of preventing unwanted pregnancies. Condoms are distributed through key contacts among the red light workers. Some come to the drop-in center and collect a week's supply. This way about 3000 condoms are disbursed every month. TENAGANITA also helps sex workers to get STD treatment. According to a social worker, "At the government clinic, preference is given to male patients. Females, on the other hand, are ridiculed and shouted at or scolded. We take patients personally and use private contacts with doctors so that they are treated better."

PINK TRIANGLE

This NGO programme of safe sex education is conducted through camps for small groups of about 10 sex workers, usually lasting three days and held every three months. The objective is to address their various needs including knowledge about HIV/AIDS, STDs and other relevant issues. Explaining the nature of training, a social worker says, "We identify girls who are natural leaders, who are vocal and liked by other girls, and take them to seaside resorts. It is very popular among them since it is the kind of 'holiday' they cannot usually afford. We also ensure that there are no men around to distract them. Workshops are conducted on empowerment: the idea of telling the client "no" is something new to them. Some clients being very rough we tell them, 'Just learn to say no. Do not allow anyone to do to your body what you don't like.'

"Rights over their body is a new concept they are teaching themselves. They know tricks about how to make the client ejaculate faster or how to put on the condom without the client's knowledge. Guest speakers talk about the sex worker's rights when they get picked up or raped by police. We also get them to develop a questionnaire on needs or AIDS knowledge and they supply their answers. We deal with health issues also; the issues which come up during outreach work are also discussed. Pubic lice is a common problem for girls. Another problem is the use of Savlon, Dettol, Guiness Stout or brandy for douching. They think it saves them from STD if they do so. We explain how it damages the lining of the vagina and also removes friendly bacteria, making them more susceptible to HIV."

The NGO is also developing a pamphlet on AIDS prevention using the language of the sex workers, avoiding scientific jargon. It plans to expand its activities to massage parlours and karoke lounges which also have sex workers. MSMs also need interventions as they have problems of poverty and unemployment. STD treatment-facilities for sex workers is another need because of discrimination against them at government clinics; and they cannot easily afford the drugs.

Although empowerment of sex workers is the long-term goal, many obstacles remain. Transsexuals have their own informal organization but cannot get it registered due to objections from the government's Religious Committee whose approval is required.

Patterns of mutual help for funerals and other social needs were developed to a considerable extent until the organization broke up due to internal rivalries. There still remains some unity, at least among those who are living in one area. In terms of empowerment, the most disadvantaged are female sex workers.

THAI RED CROSS SOCIETY

This NGO has no on-going programme of self-help activity among sex workers.

EMPOWER

The NGO's primary goal is the empowerment of sex workers. This is seen as a precondition to protect themselves and their health, including protection from HIV infection. It approaches sex workers as people rather than a category at risk of getting or giving HIV. In this respect, its attitude to sex workers is distinct from other NGOs. The director outlines its philosophy thus: "People ask me; 'Have you changed any women?'. I say: 'I am sorry, we have not. We respect people, and try to share common ideas and feelings. When we share ideas I find I am myself being changed'. Speaking of sex workers, she adds "They want a happy family and their children to have education. Their dreams are no different from our own. It is hard to change people's attitudes and make them realize that these are people and not just prostitutes."

In the last three years, more than 3000 sex workers have benefitted from self help activities initiated by EMPOWER through three outreach centers, one each at Pat Pong and Sukumvit in Bangkok and one in Chiang Mai district. NGO personnel refer to the beneficiaries as "students" with the tenor of educational emphasis very clear. The students form their own councils and committees to draw up their own policies and programmes. Two types of programmes are conducted: one is for women who are sfree to leave their workplace and come and study at the center, the other involves taking the programme to the brothels and for women who are not free to leave them. Of the two, the latter has been limited to visiting the girls and giving them condoms. Occasionally, groups go inside the brothels and clean up the place.

Programmes for non-brothel girls are conducted in the afternoons which is convenient for practically all the women. The in-house activities include language classes in Thai and English. Sewing, typing, and maths are taught mostly by Thai volunteers who are paid a travelling allowance. English is taught by foreign volunteers who are available in Thailand for about six months at a time. The classes are small and held in one large room at fixed hours and days. Many students are not Thai speaking; but speak a regional Thai dialect or are Chinese or Burmese. Most of the bar owners are foreigners and most women cater to deal with foreign guests. Sometimes girls also maintain correspondence with foreign boyfriends. Learning English has much practical value in negotiating both with owners as well as customers. About 20 sex workers attend classes each day.

The NGO also has a drama group which stages skits on safe sex and condom use at bars or in the streets. After the drama, the actors distribute free condoms to the men present. The Coordinator comments; "It is a simple drama. The message is: no matter who you are and what profession you practice or how clean you are; you can get any disease and give it to another. We have eight workshops a year for the play, recruiting new people from the streets or from a bar. It is made up of short skits with no dialogue. The actors use mime, songs, whistles, and other props. Dialogues are not used as the message will be lost, the area being very noisy; and the women are not professional actors. In every center, they have a different kind of drama.

"In all education programmes there is a health and AIDS component. Health workshops are held once about every two months. There are also group counselling sessions where women share experiences and health problems, how to cope, how to get treatment, and doctors seen.

"Other sessions focus on daily problems and dealing with them; such as how to open a bank account, operate a cash machine, write a letter, and have translations of letters from foreign boy friends. Earlier they used to put cash in an envelope and send it home; now they know how to fill Money Order forms. Even when they fell sick, they didn't even have the confidence to explain their problem to a doctor.

"That is self-empowerment—to know who they are and to study themselves; to be with a group and know to do things together. We had legal workshops last year for every center. Women want to know more about the law now. We would not acheive this kind of participation had we organized a meeting with a lawyer for them. Nobody would want to see a lawyer unless we start from a group counselling situation. They talk, and whenever problems come up we find books on law for them.

"The NGO has also started non-formal education programmes for sex workers who had left school at an early age. At present there are 73 students with eight at the high school level, 20 in the secondary school and the rest in primary."

EMPOWER also holds conferences for sex workers. As the Coordinator says, "After they come to the center they become confident. Most of these women come from the countryside and don't know how to get around in the city usually commuting by taxi or motorcycle (if they are bar workers). We take them on tours to science museums, printing factories, shoe and clothes factories, palaces and printing shops. This year, we are taking some to meet the sex workers in the government rehabilitation center. We build confidence in the students on how to organize programmes. A camp is also held outside Bangkok for one night".

It also has an outreach publication in the form of a newsletter which is distributed free describing its programmes, health issues, the AIDS situation and women's issues such as abortion.

The process of empowerment is slow but sure and consists of building survival skills. An example of this was demonstrated recently when sex workers took to the streets protesting a government proposal to extend business hours of bars till 3.00 a.m. They would never have dreamed of something like this in the past.

EMPOWER's attempts to promote self help among sex workers are limited due to its small resources, obtained from abroad, and no support from the Thai government. In Pat Pong area, for example, the target population is more than 5000 women of which they have reached only 3000 during the last 10 years.

The Coordinator adds "Many of them are scattered around now and work in Phuket or Pataya. Some have married and settled down while others have gone abroad. Before they leave, they come and inform us so that we send them materials and copies of the newsletter. Some even help us in disseminating the work we do."

The NGO sees empowerment of sex workers as part and parcel of a larger process of social change needed in Thai society. In the words of the Coordinator: "We still have a long way to go in terms of society's attitude to women, in terms of the government's way of solving their problems which is trying to impose things. We are working as a medium of communication between the sex worker and other agents. One way of getting their act together is by voicing their problems. We tell them if they participate in elections, their votes will count. The mass media helped a lot, making the public more aware of them.

People started understanding them as women and not simply as prostitutes"

ACCESS

The NGO has not focussed its attention on self help initiatives among sex workers excepting condom promotion in brothels in Chiang Mai district, started two years ago.

CFPA

Self help initiatives for sex workers in Sri Lanka's Southern province began in September 1994 with the recruitment and training of six peer educators. This included a husband and wife team (from Dondra) who worked as pimps, and four ex-beach boys, two each from Batigama and Hikkaduwa who were 'community leaders' in their respective villages. The author, as a programme manager, visited potential recruits at their homes and reinforced the importance of their participation in intervention work and the need to gain more knowledge about the work itself. CFPA was to pay them a monthly allowance of Rs 500 once they were recruited after training. A three-day residential workshop was held for the team at the outreach center in Hikkaduwa. The workshop was inaugurated by the trainees themselves, each lighting a small clay oil lamp. They were also given an opportunity to express themselves by drawing self portraits using crayons and pencil, making short speeches about themselves and their lives, performing dramatic skits, and making their own AIDS posters.

Trainers, including the team of counsellors, also took part in the training. They participated in the same exercises, ate the same food, and sat on the same mats along with the trainees. Informal discussions on STD, HIV/AIDS, safe sex practices, and prevention strategies of other Asian NGOs took place during the second and third days of training. Although discussions were led by people with expertise in their relevant fields, trainees were encouraged to ask questions and re-interpret technical terms in their own social and terminological contexts.

On several occasions, trainers had to face embarrassment when trainees used colloquial terms to describe sex, types of sex acts, and parts of the human anatomy. Conversely, trainees had to come to terms with difficult technical jargon such as “HIV”, “STD”, “safe sex”, and “counselling”.

They were also given demonstrations of proper condom use and disposal using wooden penile models on which they practiced individually. A small supply of free condoms was given before they left for their homes and photographs taken for issuing them identity cards. Within a couple of months two female sex workers, one from Galle and another from Hikkaduwa, were recruited after a short orientation progrmme. The aim was to increase access to the female sex worker population there.

The effectiveness of the peer educator model as a tool for enhancing trust through empowerment and education was amply demonstrated in the next three months. The husband and wife team from Dondra had converted their home into an AIDS and STD inforrmation center arid put up their own signboard to that effect. An entire wall of the living room was covered with hand-drawn posters and AIDS prevention messages and paraphernalia for the benefit of customers and visitors.

Meanwhile, the team of peer educators from Hikkaduwa planned to use a cadjan hut along the beach as an AIDS information booth and informal counselling center for beach boys; who used to socialize in it earlier.

Other areas in which self help initiatives were promoted by CFPA included education about STDs through a handbook giving symptoms to look out for, helping in obtaining treatment for STDs at government clinics, providing free condoms for distribution among peers, and promoting participation in programme activities such as World AIDS day events including poster competitions. In the subsequent months, seeing the success of the first group, plans were under way to recruit a second batch of peer educators.

VI. FEASIBILITY OF SAFE SEX AMONG SEX WORKERS

The promotion of safe sex, meaning the use of condoms with every penetrative sexual act, is no easy task in the situations surveyed due to a variety of interrelated factors including.

(a) Lack of education among most sex workers.
(b) Subordinate position of females vis-a-vis males.
(c) Presence of language barriers between educators and sex workers.
(d) Lack of awareness about the nature of HIV and STD among sex workers, including general indifference to health and sanitation.
(e) The nature of the sex act itself; which usually takes place without conversation, the idea being to have sex as quickly as possible, leaving little opportunity for negotiation.
(f) The lack of awareness among customers about the nature of HIV and STD, particularly if they are from the ranks of blue collar workers and other socially underprivileged groups.
(g) Lack of organization among sex workers, so that if one refuses to have sex without condoms, the customers will always find another one willing.
(h) Unwillingness of sex workers to have condoms with them especially in situations where carrying condoms can lead to police arrest or where the sex worker is unwilling to go to a store and buy her own condoms.
(i) The type of context in which sex takes place; which may be a dingy room or a public park or a similar place not conducive to either negotiate condom use or even wear one.
(j) Inability to do close monitoring of safe sex promotion, and
(k) The disproportional nature of the quantum of NGO intervention in relation to the number of sex workers to be covered in a particular context.

The above conclusions could be arrived at through field observations and comments of NGO officials surveyed were as follows:

IHO

With about 200 peer educators and five social workers, IHO managed to ensure free disposal of condoms to nearly 7000 sex workers in about four large brothels in central Bombay. This constitutes about four per cent of the estimated population of 175,000 sex workers in the city. Even working among this relatively small number, IHO had to overcome language barriers due to the fact that many sex workers hail from other states or countries especially Nepal. In such cases the dangers of HIV and STD was communicated through photo albums focusing on the advantages of condom use; including prevention of STD, cutting down health care costs, prevention of unwanted pregnancies, and saving money to send to dependants. Evidence suggested that the condoms disbursed weekly through the peer educators were in fact being used. Though monitored through regular discussions with peer educators and staff, there is no guarantee of hundred per cent condom use.

In brothels, sex usually takes place within a matter of six to ten minutes, and in small crowded cubicles. Despite these obstacles, safe sex practices are actively promoted by peers educators. Some sex workers however complained about losing business because of condoms, and talking about AIDS: customers think that the sex worker has it. A *saheli* had done role plays in the brothel itself and educated sex workers about how to negotiate with clients. If the customer did not want to put on the condom, the girls put it on for them, making safe sex a feasible proposition.

IHO's director sounds equally optimistic when he says, "We did sero testing of two groups, an experimental group using condoms and a control group not using them. In the former, the incidence of HIV within a period of two years rose from 32 in the preceding year to 44 in the ensuing year. In the control group, the incidence was 60 per cent." He is certain that the success rate will be higher among groups where the peer educator model is at work. At the moment it is close to 90 per cent. The balance 10 per cent is attributed to women who do not use condoms when having sex or to partners who are not faithful. There are also women who want to get pregnant and therefore do not use condoms when having sex with their boyfriends.

Sex workers in Bombay, as in most parts of the world, are not unionized. They cannot demand "No sex without condoms!" Moreover, those who use condoms are small in number, and a customer not willing to use them can always find a willing partner.

The crux of the problem is not the sex worker alone; safe sex will simply not be possible on a significant scale without the cooperation of the customers. As the director of *Prerna,* an NGO seeking to uplift conditions of sex workers in Bombay, said "Women are not so empowered that they can get a man to use condoms. They can bargain only with regular customers or those willing to use them. Dumping condoms on them is not going to help: In fact women react negatively when this is done. Only 10 per cent will use condoms and they may not even use it for every sexual act, especially with their boyfriends or regular partners."

GAP

GAP's experience with sex workers is still in the trial stages. With some intervention activity having commenced in Surat's red light area, it sees unionization as a prerequisite for making safe sex feasible and sustainable. In the words of GAP's director: "I am working to get them together, to form their own union, give them solidarity and let them understand (the danger) so that a day will come when all of them will say 'we are all using condoms.' When they say 'we use condoms', it means so once in a while and not for every encounter. If there is hundred per cent use, in one month there should be 150 to 200 condoms used by one person, which means 1500 to 2000 condoms per house. In that case there should be a mountain of (used) condoms!"

She sees the problem as one arising from the inferior status of women which reduces their ability to negotiate. One social worker in Surat added the monetary dimension: "If the man gives more money, he dominates the relationship. At the same time, the insistence of Hindu sex workers on only vaginal sex places them at greater risk. Also, women have their own methods for determining whether sex with a particular customer is safe or not. If a man is unclean in the genital area, they will not have sex with him."

Attitudes among sex workers to their profession is a contributory factor for not having safe sex. Says the social worker, "When this lady told me she had customers who were coming drunk, I told her, 'You may not go in for vaginal sex. Why not use other methods like masturbation'? Her answer was 'It is not right to do so' since she would have already taken money from him (for vaginal sex). However, the shock treatment appears to have helped in certain instances.

Recalling another experience with a sex worker, the social worker said "I told one lady, 'If you want to be in this business, don't you think you have to be physically fit? You have to start protecting yourself. If you don't use condoms, you are likely to go through it (AIDS).' I don't know whether it was right to frighten her, but she started using condoms." However, some girls are virtually unapproachable, especially those from Nepal who do not communicate and prefer to remain withdrawn.

CAN

This NGO is somewhat unique, believing that condom use would be ensured if sex workers bought it or got their clients to buy it from them or their brokers. The logic is, "If any client can pay 300 rupees for sex, he is not going to hesitate to buy a condom." This policy, however, applies to female sex workers only, whereas transsexuals and MSMs get them free of cost. Furthermore, since CAN disburs,es *Delux Nirodh* instead of the ordinary monocoloured variety, it believes that clients and even sex workers will be motivated to buy or use them. One official asserted, "We have Fiesta condoms which are see-through and colorful. It has a fancy element and is attractive, better lubricated and of better quality, and easily available in the market."

Whether all this ensures that a client will purchase condoms from either the prostitution network or the open market is open to question. CAN has a dual monitoring system; one being daily reports from social workers as to how many condoms-were distributed among the peer educators, and another independent team which regularly gets report from clients. It is doubtful whether such a monitoring team will have access to either female sex workers or their clients given the secretive nature of prostitution in general. More particularly in the case of female sex workers who operate entirely in secret. Again, given the large number of sex workers and clients in Madras, and even in the selected intervention sites, such a team could only do spot checks on a random basis.

CAN officials are however optimistic. As one puts it: "The women are responsible and want to take preventive action. The men are at greater fault: they have the money and are drunk; all they want to do is to have sex. The women should take the responsibility of always using condoms. They are completely rational and are concerned about their health. In some brothels, women read newspapers while having sex. They can think of other things even when having sex."

Is there any negotiation involved in using condoms'? CAN officials feel it depends on the sex worker's background and the extent to which she regards her work as a profession. "Negotiating condom use is always in the hands of the sex worker and depends on how good she is at her job. Women who come from the temple *(devdasi)* system have very few taboos regarding sex and have been successful in getting their clients to use condoms. They respect their bodies, always having a bath, and getting their client to take a bath, before having sex. They also first serve food to the client; and are in control of the situation. We have begun to think that sex work should be professionalised."

This observation gives an interesting dimension to the feasibility of safe sex. Merely pushing condom use is thus not going to ensure their use. Negotiation skills have to be placed in the context of sex work, including not only where and how it takes place but also the attitude of the sex worker to clients, and to the work she is doing.

SIAAP

SIAAP's Director believes that safe sex is feasible, and hundred per cent condom use can be ensured. But a series of obstacles exist and removing them will take time and effort. The obstacles were identified as:

(a) Putting the safe sex message in a broader context than HIV, and in relation to the whole person of WIPs ('women in prostitution' which SIAAP prefers to "sex worker"). In her words: "We have to approach women with a concern for their care. We don't need to worry about what is happening to the world with HIV, and instead approach the women with a personal concern. In doing so we should be able to explain the situation of AIDS in the context of her reality, and how it is going to affect her lifestyle. Not merely in relation to illness, since she may not even get the virus, but what it will do to the community of which she is a part. That is why community organization is so important." Concern can be communicated to a sex worker in the following terms: "You owe it to yourself to protect yourself, and we will be able to provide you with some form of consistent support."

(b) Negotiation is done at two levels: negotiating with clients, and accessing the condoms. Elaborating on these SIAAP's director states, "Earlier people were saying that women will not be able to tell a client and demand condom use, and many more women never attempted to negotiate. We did not teach them to negotiate. All we did was explain to them the risk. We demonstrated how a condom should be used (using an improvised and less conspicuous penile model than the one conventionally used). Then we asked them how they were going to tell the client, and they came up with six or seven different ways which they started trying. They have more skills than one could dream of".

Psychological empowerment is seen as an indispensable basis for negotiating with condoms. The Director's message to the sex worker is: "You are often seen by society either as fallen victims, or at worst, as sinners or criminals. Both are positions of utter powerlessness. You cannot hope to function in a position of powerlessness. We believe you are in a position of power. Why? Because despite everything that has happened to you—rape, being sold, etc.—today you earn a livelihood. You support other people.

Day after day, despite the brutalization you have gone through, you stand there, you look good, you have poise. You have so much strength that you are back on the streets. Are you telling me you are not strong? Are you not strong to use a condom? You are strong in the friendships you have. If a lover walks out on you, then you have another. In the real world, you are strong women. Don't let other people tell you that you are weak. Are you not strong enough to stop a man from killing you simply because he is so silly as to have sex without a condom?".

She does admit to practical difficulties when negotiation takes place. One problem is when clients think the WIP must be having some disease, otherwise why should she ask him to wear a condom. Secondly, the WIP must be convinced about what she is suggesting to the client. If convinced, she believes that negotiation will be hundred per cent effective. Thirdly, the women must be prepared to put on the condom for the man. SIAAP has been able to persuade WIPs to overcome the reluctance to handle a man's penis. It becomes a chore for the man and "chances of the condom getting used will be more if the women put it on for the men."

Fourthly, some conditions favour condom use particularly when the man has no option but to put on a condom: "In some places, the man has given the money. He has taken off his clothes and is sitting with an erection. The condom is on the table; and she takes it and starts putting it on him. Although he has the option of not putting on one, the situation is such that nine out of ten men will not walk out." One of SIAAP's social workers explains that younger WIP's have a better chance of practicing safe sex methods than older ones: "Younger women are more willing to participate in the programme. They read some literature and are active and more smart, less fatalistic, and more receptive. Besides, they can always get more clients if one refuses to have sex with a condom."

The second factor is accessing condoms, and here SIAAP's outlook is radically different from that of CAN which believes that sex workers and clients should be asked to pay for condoms. In the Director's view such an approach is based on a lack of understanding of the realities of commercial sex; at least in the South Indian context. "These women, usually coming from low income backgrounds, are not psychologically conditioned for going to a shop. Shops come to them; whether it is clothes or cosmetics they rarely go out. Besides, there is a cultural stigma attached to prostitution; in a brothel area it may be different.

"In a street worker situation, it becomes twice as difficult for a woman to go to a shop and ask for a condom. She is supposed to be anonymous. The social perception is that if any woman goes to a shop and asks for a condom, she is a prostitute. That itself is a big barrier for condom use even for ordinary people. Besides, the WIP herself has a nagging feeling of guilt that she is doing something wrong, that she is living in sin and has to be hidden every day. The whole world is telling her that; and she lives on the brink of sanity. The inner world of WIPs is so different from others. The world outside has become more oppressive towards WIPs. Since the advent of HIV police oppression has increased. For the last 10 years, the government has run ad campaigns saying 'Don't go to prostitutes ! ' The perception is that these women are spreading AIDS.'

In such a context, social marketing is misplaced and also seen as counter-productive. "It may be relevant if the world allows a woman to walk into a shop and ask for condoms, if the client cooperates, and if the brothel keeper really cares about the women. But the brothel keepers are like drug pushers; it is a business for them. If they lose one woman today, another will walk in tomorrow. In addition women cannot carry condoms around; they tried, and were arrested for it." The pressure from donors to promote social marketing is seen, quite rightly, at least from the street worker's angle, as unethical. "They will support free immunization, but will not support free condoms because it revolves around sex. Condoms have been given for family planning for the last 40 years, but now for HIV they cannot."

Unavailability of good quality condoms through government sources is another disadvantage. The Director recalls sending them for quality tests which they failed, forcing SIAAP to purchase deluxe *Nirodh* from the open market, the monthly bill for which is around two lakh rupees. She added with a gesture of despair, "How can we run a programme like that?" Ensuring that good quality condoms are within easy reach of the WIPs has been a central goal of SIAAP. A first step was to get the cooperation of lodge (hotel) owners and make an appeal to their good sense. "We called them together and said, 'This is a small thing for you (to keep condoms at the lodge); can you imagine saving people's lives? How many have the power to do that?' It touched a chord; to do some good."

I sincerely believe that people feel the need to do good but just do not know how to go about it. A little effort and people immediately respond. "Some complained that they might be liable to police arrest if they kept condoms. We explained to them the purpose of keeping condoms and having a room boy deliver it with the traditional glass of water when a client comes with a female. Keeping it on the table so that the woman does not have to negotiate on it. The idea was that she should not have to put extra effort (to make the condom a part of the whole sex scenario), knowing that she has so many other stresses negotiating with clients and the outside world, and with illness." Some hotel owners would try to sell the condoms given by SIAAP or wait till the women came and asked for them.

Constant persuasion and monitoring through the counsellors and by the Director herself is an on-going process. Daily reports of field staff giving details of how many condoms were given and in what place are followed by checks with lodge owners. (The NGO's 18 peer educators and two female field workers are not able to come to the main office regularly but have to be met in the field.) Tracking of all WIPs with regard to actual condom use is not practically possible. And the number of condoms disbursed remains the main criteria for monitoring; with nearly 9000 of them directly distributed by SIAAP in Madras city alone. However, SIAAP has been working with three other NGOs in the city, two of which it still funds. Including them the total condoms distributed every month in Madras comes to about 50,000 pieces.

In a sense, SIAAP's activities unwittingly complement those of CAN which does not cover female sex workers in Madras. The present coverage, however, is limited only to a sixth of the population, and that too without adequate means of delivering safe sex services to them.

TENAGANITA

Although condoms are handed out to sex workers, the NGO does not appear to be conducting any monitoring of their use.

PINK TRIANGLE

The issue of empowerment has been its key concern. It sees empowerment as being directly proportional to safe sex practices adopted by sex workers. A social worker recalls how "All 30 girls in one hotel decided to use condoms, while earlier it depended on the whim and fancy of the client. Now, if the client refuses, the girl gets her pimp to persuade the client and bring him round to agree." However, as is illustrated, agreement among sex workers is by itself not a sufficient condition. The cooperation and some impetus from the hierarchy of prostitution is also necessary.

Obstacles to safe sex also emanate from two other sources: drug abuse among sex workers, and the nature of the client. As another social worker commented, "Women who take to drugs and are high on it or having withdrawal symptoms, will not think of safe sex." The initiative always comes back to the client even though most girls agree to use condoms. For instance, if the client does not agree, the girl fails to insist otherwise, fearing that the man will beat her. Very often the men do not use condoms because they "would not be getting their money's worth." On the other hand, if say a woman's husband has been arrested for drugs, and she needs money to support her children, HIV is a remote consideration.

Other habits of drug users are a further obstacle. "They take a shot and move elsewhere as a result of which they cannot spend time at the drop-in center. Safe sex education has to be persistent. And such persistent education is not possible given the limited resources of the NGO and lack of staff. P.T depends on the reports of five of its outreach workers. The problems they face daily are talked about and documented; and as needs come up they are addressed. Another necessary condition is self esteem of the sex worker. A social worker says "Any harm reduction method will work only if the girls have developed self esteem. Otherwise they believe that society has rejected them."

The NGO supplies condoms and encourages sex workers to buy them once they have started using them regularly. Of the 1500 target population in the Chowkit area, it has promoted condom use (not 100 per cent) among 300 sex workers. Negotiating skills have also been imparted, including use of oral sex in place of anal sex among transsexuals. One social worker's advice to sex workers was, "Tell the client that if he uses a condom, you will feel fine. Tell him you can come even when he uses condoms. Men are often worried that the girl may not be enjoying herself if they (men) wear a condom. Explain that the condom is used not because you don't trust him but because: 'Your wife will not know you are having sex with me if you use a condom. This way no one will know that you have been having sex outside. On the other hand, if you get infected your wife will get to know.' I also tell the sex worker that she will have to spend more money for STD treatment if she does not protect herself."

Another practical obstacle is the fear of being raided by the police. On how this affects negotiation, the social worker says, "With frequent police raids taking place, sex workers do not want to take much time to negotiate condom use with clients. And without the time they cannot explain things to clients. But it is easier if sex is taking place in their own house or apartment." Thus, the context in which sex takes place is an important factor.

THAI RED CROSS SOCIETY

Two pilot interventions in gay bars carried out by G.Carl, the counsellor, provide an important perspective to the problem of promoting safe sex through condom use. It was found that as Iong as condoms were brought by the counsellor and given to the male sex workers they were willing to use them. Consequently, incidence of HIV and Hepatitis B among them remained low. But when the supply was no longer available this way, condom use dropped. The counsellor recalled how one manager came to his office asking him to bring condoms rather than getting them himself as he (the manager) was too shy. The manager was not even keen enough to send one of the boys to do it. Given the cultural stigma attached to obtaining condoms, the responsibility for not only promoting safe sex but also supplying condoms falls on the change agent. In this context, the SIAAP director's observations on social marketing are valid for Asian society as a whole, where social taboos regarding condom purchasing hold for males as well.

Social expectations from the two sexes are a further dimension of the problem. Says G.C, "Society views a woman carrying condoms with suspicion. Condom use for birth control is acceptable since it has more to do with economics. But when it comes to sexual gratification it becomes another story. Already it is the woman's responsibility to practice birth control and the same attitude should prevail for protecting herself against HIV. What do the men do then? In Thai culture, like in most of Asia, women are supposed to be concerned about reproduction and men about sexual gratification. A lot of women tolerate husbands going to sex workers saying, 'I have my family, a house, and what I need socially. Why do I need him or his sexual urges?' There is little negotiation between sexual partners. Communication has broken down. Alliances are common outside marriage. Some women even say, 'It is better he has sex with sex workers than with a minor wife (a concubine), which is an economic responsibility.' There is tacit acceptance; and the real need is for empowerment of women, not after, but before marriage."

Most female sex workers appear to bargain from a position of social inequality vis-a-vis male clients, and apparently, this determines the outcome of negotiation. As a counsellor at the Red Cross observed: "It is difficult to get men to wear condoms because they are mostly drunk when going to a sex worker. They will have the condom in the pocket but will not use it. They would rather go to the girl who wants money and does not make an issue of condoms. Most girls are afraid of losing money." In addition, lack of awareness among women, that anyone could be an HIV carrier, prevents them from insisting on condom use. Some girls look at the appearance of men, and if they are well-dressed or talk nicely, they are considered to be free of infection. People who are dirty are thought to be infected.

The policy of each establishment also has a role in promoting safe sex. In Pataya, for instance, if the male sex worker refuses to work without condoms, the bar will compensate him for the time lost. And yet there are others who will say that the customer is always right.

What then of the claim that there is hundred per cent condom use in some parts of Thailand? G.C. is extremely skeptical when he says, "The safe sex campaigns conducted by the government are not all that effective. It is typical of Thais to say: 'The campaign is a success; we can stop now.' The campaign was conducted in one or two-provinces by supplying condoms to sex workers, giving them condom education, and health officers doing surveillance checks. The sex workers were required to go to the clinic for STD and HIV examinations. If they found any incidence of STD, they were given a warning the first time. If they found it again, the bar was closed down for a day, and if yet again, for three days, and then permanently. Overall, condom use registered was about 30 per cent. If the campaign was working as claimed, it would shoot up to 98 per cent. I asked 'If we have hundred per cent condom use, why do we have so many clients with STD in our clinic?' Also, the information gathered was through interviews. Sex workers are asked: 'Do you use condoms? How often?' The sex worker, knowing that saying "no" will invite a lecture, says "yes" all the time. It is a threatening interview process."

G.C. believes that the solution is more complicated and demanding: "The campaign is generally conducted by a truckload of health workers who go into a bar and say, 'OK; this is what you have to do, etc., and then leave. They need someone who is an inhouse counsellor, someone who gets to know their needs, really talks to them; not as a health worker or a client. Having peer educators in bars is not easy. You can get sex workers who are trained, but negative peer pressure (among sex workers) is always there. In some bars, where older sex workers undergo some health education, the new ones do not have many questions to ask and then someone will always say: "Well, we have heard this before; let's get to work". If someone is there as a friend and a counsellor and explains things face to face, is supportive, and also has the supply and delivery of condoms on time, then there will be results."

Differential status among health worker and sex worker is seen as an inhibiting factor. "The health workers are way up there and the sex workers are down below in terms of social status. Somehow, to elevate these people, the talking has to be more on equal terms. The easiest thing is for the health worker to come down."

EMPOWER

The NGO has no condom promotion campaign and lays emphasis on empowerment of sex workers. The logic is that once empowerment takes place safe sex practices would automatically follow along with an increased ability to negotiate condom use with clients. At present, the NGO's activities with regard to condoms include (a) free distribution of condoms to sex workers who attend training programmes, workshops and seminars (b) staging a play with safe sex messages in three locations once a month and (c) free distribution of gift-wrapped condoms among customers after the skits on condoms and AIDS are performed.

EMPOWER does not believe in the concept of peer educators or using them to educate sex workers about safe sex or to deliver condoms. The Coordinator mentioned that there were more men using condoms now than four or five years ago, and that at the moment their primary concern was not AIDS prevention. He added: "Using condoms is a problem everywhere. Women do not have the power to force a man to wear one. Everybody knows they are at risk. Some bars and brothels support such women. But, if the women refuse customers, they will lose money." In other words, safe sex depends on the whim and fancy of the customer and the policy of the brothel or bar management. There is no indication that positive attitudes to condom use are emerging on any significant scale either among customers or managements. In that sense, the picture is extremely bleak.

ACCESS

The experience of this NGO with safe sex promotion among female sex workers, although limited in scope, has some useful lessons. When their field staff approached the sex workers in Chiang Mai, they (sex workers) said that so many different organizations had come to them and talked about safe sex that they were willing to use condoms. According to the Director, although the local public health office provided them with condoms, "The problem was with the customers." Attempts to educate the customers were not rewarding: "We would talk to them before they went in. Some were drunk and could hardly be talked to. Others would harass the female members of our team." The key factor was the push given by the brothel owners who had formed an association and were aware of HIV. "They had all agreed to put up notices for the customers asking them to use condoms. Before that they were not using condoms at all. When our team made a survey after the new rules came, it was found that 40 per cent clients used condoms after this course of action."

What made these brothel owners different? Was it simple concern about protecting the workers from HIV? The scale of the brothel operation and ties with the sex workers based on regional identity and kinship were key co-factors. "In northern Thailand, the brothel owners are local people. They are small business people and the relationship between them and the sex workers is quite good. It is more like a family relationship and sometimes they are related by kinship." These crucial factors are missing in the large brothels of Bangkok where the sex workers have been supplied by brokers and are managed purely for financial gain. The numbers are too large for managers to develop good relationships with them or be concerned about their health. Lack of unions among owners further contributes to competition among them and thus the absence of a clear stand or policy regarding condom use for customers.

CFPA

The NGO began promoting safe sex through condom use by recruiting the first batch of peer educators. Their task was to deliver condoms to peers and/or customers and keep a record of how many condoms were given, and how consistently they were used by those receiving them. Each peer educator was given a handbook containing pictures showing correct use of condoms. The field staff would visit the peer educators once every two weeks, monitor the progress made, and find out whether more condoms were needed. All monitoring activities were reviewed once every two weeks when the field staff met the programme coordinator. Obstacles to condom promotion came from several sources:

(a) Supply of quality condoms

The first supply of condoms were obtained free of charge through WHO's AIDS Project office in Colombo. Feedback from peer educators revealed that the condoms were definitely better than *preethi,* the cheapest condom brand available in the market, one which was also promoted for family planning. Users of the new condom had found them to be better lubricated and, unlike *preethi,* free of the rubber-like smell. Besides, there was an additional (social) value to the new condom since it was "foreign made" and packed in attractive blue or purple colours.

Unfortunately, as their demand increased, the supply was not sufficient and regular enough due to procedural delays. An adequate stock was made available only in January 1995, five months after the peer educator programme had commenced. As a result monitoring of condom use was hampered from September 1994 to January 1995. To meet the exigency some peer educators had to purchase condoms at their own expense, but given their low income level, it is unlikely that they were able to meet the demand.

(b) Accessing Condoms

Since peer educators kept the condoms in their homes or at some other convenient point, those wishing to use them were spared the embarrassment of going to a shop; a problem common to both men and women in Sri Lanka as in other Asian countries. Again, unlike pharmacies and small grocery shops, which serve as commercial condoms outlets, the users could obtain condoms from the peer educator at any time of the day, or night particularly, when business establishments are closed.

This facility was all the more beneficial to female sex workers who chose to have condoms with them when picked up by a customer. A female peer educator from Hikkaduwa recalls: "When a girl arrives in town she has no money to spare, having left home with only the bus fare. As money is usually paid after sex, she is unable to go to a shop and buy condoms. And most shops are closed by the time a girl gets a customer. But as I live near the town it is very convenient for them. After picking up a customer girls ask him to wait till she gets free condoms from me".

(c) Keeping a tab on use and users

When peer educators were asked to keep a record of who used how many condoms and how often, it created a problem. They came from a cultural system in which keeping a close tab on behavioral details was neither the norm nor did it have any value. In the subculture of poverty to which they belonged, maintaining accounts of anything was an irrelevant activity: they lived from day to day, spending all they had earned by the end of the evening. They were not used to keeping records of any kind. Some were not literate, having only had a primary education. There was no way they could be re-socialized into the middle class values of the change agent. One possible option was to recruit a literate and somewhat educated member. This is only hindsight, and an option that was not explored.

(d) Cooperation of Brothel Managers

By December 1994, two women peer educators had made contact with girls working in a couple of brothels, each having about 10 girls. The demand for condoms was much higher for this sector as opposed to the small numbers required by the street girls. A female sex worker who was the key contact in one brothel had suggested that she be given at least 100 condoms a day. But at that stage in the programme, delivery of large stocks could not be possible without the explicit consent of the management which operated secretly. The next logical step was to obtain their cooperation, but it is not known whether the field staff were successful in doing so.

(e) Availability of Lubricants

Some sex workers, particularly females, had complained to the peer educators of vaginal irritation after sex and believed this to be a symptom of STD or a result of using condoms. Once they were free of such infection by getting tested at a clinic, it was found to be a result of not using lubricants. Using recommended lubricants, the difficulty was overcome. The above fact makes it clear that once people were made sufficiently aware of the health benefits of condom use they were quite willing to adopt them.

But this does not end the process of intervention since sustaining it is a shared responsibility involving both change agents as well as the intended beneficiaries. It would be correct to say that this responsibility lies more with the former than with the latter. In the first place, the change agent has to develop a carefully thought out strategy covering all aspects of intervention. This should include taking into account probable obstacles and how to overcome them even before giving out the message of safe sex. Typically, most NGOs fail in this respect relying more on hindsight or, at best, trial and error. The delays and confusions that result could be costly from the viewpoint of controlling the epidemic.

VII. CORRIDORS AND LINKS WITH POVERTY

Here the routes of transmission or corridors and the links between socioeconomic factors such as poverty, migration and prostitution are discussed.

1. CORRIDORS

Links between prostitution and transport and other corridors pertain mainly to overland routes such as highways and bridges connecting cities or countries. These serve as corridors both for sex workers to migrate from one city or country to another, and for prospective customers to have access to sex workers.

Examples from the study are as follows:

Gujarat (India)

Trucks entering or leaving the city of Ahmedabad halt overnight for loading or unloading operations at several stations including Aslali Nagar and Chendula Nagar. There are between 500 to 1000 trucks parked every night at these stations. And every truck has a driver and a cleaner. At each such station prostitution is common. The crew travels from one city to another for a period of about 15 days after which they return to their villages; most of them coming from Rajasthan.

A large number of migrant labour also come from Rajasthan and Andhra Pradesh to work in the construction companies of Ahmedabad. They include men and women from rural areas who come to earn some money after the planting of crops in their native villages is over. They return to their villages for the harvesting season when their labour is required. The construction labourers working in Surat are mostly from Orissa state and live in the city's low income enclaves.

Maharashtra (India)

The main corridors are express highways, including the Eastern Highway connecting Bombay with Julwaniya in Madhya Pradesh, and the Western Highway to Hyderabad, Bangalore and Goa. Bus stops and railway stations are points for prostitution. Bombay also has two international ports and one international airport giving easy access to people from all over the world to its red light areas.

Tamil Nadu (India)

Express highways used by long distance truck drivers form the main corridor in Tamil Nadu. Madras has a check post where all trucks plying north to south (Tamil Nadu to Orissa and Tamil Nadu to Uttar Pradesh) stop for one or two days to empty cargo and wait for the return cargo. (About two million such trucks operate all over India). Truck stops in Madras, like in most parts of India, not only provide food and shelter but also commercial sex.

Tamil Nadu also has several places of pilgrimage to which come people from all over India as well as from outside. Tirichendu, Tirupathi, Madurai, and Velangani are a few such pilgrimage centers which have hotels and lodges, and where prostitution takes place. Large crowds also gather once a year at Sonepur, in Bihar, for India's largest cattle fair. This is also an ideal locale for prostitution.

Malaysia

The movement of populations from neighbouring countries through Malaysia has been the result of rapid industrialization. It also poses a problem with regard to control of HIV in the region. In recent years, more and more people have come from across the Philippines, Indonesia, and Bangladesh for employment in the country's construction work, factories, and plantations. Most of them are migrant workers who come on contract. Without their families, these people form the main clientele for prostitution in the urban areas. Construction labourers sometimes have to work for several weeks at a stretch in distant places. And when they are free, sex becomes the main form of entertainment. They are quite mobile often moving from one location to another. Women workers who come for employment in new factories also, in their spare time, engage in prostitution for an extra income.

Access to Thailand, which has a high incidence of HIV, is another reason. Being easily approachable by road and rail, Thailand is frequented mostly through direct buses and trains operating through Penang. Most of the people go with the intention of having sex since it very cheap, the fee being as little as 30 dollars for a sex worker (A Malaysian girl would cost 10 times more). At the same time, at least two to three thousand agricultural workers come to Malaysia from Thailand to work in the rice fields; which also contributes to the spread of HIV.

Thailand

Geographical (horizontal) mobility among sex workers has been identified as a principal factor contributing to the transmission of HIV across the country. As G.C. explains, "Sex workers from the north will go to Hatyai, and then move to Bangkok, and from there to Patayai and Phuket in the south and then move to Ckiang Mai (in the north). Migration patterns played a significant role even 20 years back. There is also a transient population of agricultural labour. During the off season they also drive taxis or trucks."

Prostitution is inevitably linked with rural poverty; particularly due to low incomes from agriculture, a result of irregular water supply and the high cost of agricultural inputs. With the emphasis on industrialization, there is a glut for landless agricultural labourers some of who go and work in neighboring Malaysia.

Principal truck routes have also largely contributed to the spread of the epidemic. These are Bangkok to Chiang Mai going upto Chiang Rai, and then to Kon Ken in the lower northeast. There are routes from central Thailand to the northeast, and from there to the north. According to G.C, "The damage through these corridors has already been done". Truck drivers are known to take amphetamines (a drug prohibited in the country but available at gas stations in a small brown bottle). Mixed with caffeine and nicotine, it keeps them alert during long drives so that even when they stop for a rest, they are unable to go to sleep. They believe that the only way to bring down the high is to have sex. And that is easily done considering that many sex workers frequent truck stops.

The recent opening of Friendship Bridge connecting Thailand with Laos and Cambodia is another disaster from the viewpoint of HIV control. Because it is now possible to recruit girls, some underage, from any of these countries into the brothels of Thailand.

Sri Lanka

Patterns of HIV transmission in Sri Lanka are similar to those prevaling in other Asian countries. They include main highways diverging from the capital city of Colombo to the rural hinterland, railway routes connecting the city with other peripheral cities and towns, weekly markets, and pilgrimage centers. The nodes in these networks are invariably linked with prostitution, as many sex workers keep travelling from one point to another partly in an effort to avoid detection and arrest by law enforcers. Interestingly, statistics compiled by the government's STD control campaign show that drivers and traders form over 50 per cent of the men treated for STD at government clinics.

Labour migration to Middle Eastern and East Asian countires, particularly to Singapore, is another potential source of transmission. A large majority of migrants to these countries are females employed principally as domestic servants. Incidentally, about five known HIV cases were found to be such women who had a history of employment in the Middle East.

Sri Lanka also has two international ports and one international airport. Many Sri Lankans have also found employment as seamen in international shipping firms; and they constitute a fair number of the known HIV cases in the country.

Another population movement fraught with risk of HIV transmission has been Sri Lanka's refugee problem, an outcome of the separatist war. Nearly 30 thousand people from the north had to take refuge in Tamil Nadu, India, which also has a high incidence of HIV. They are at the moment being repatriated, and pose a real threat for HIV transmission once they settle down in Sri Lanka. This dislocation, it may be mentioned, has also led people to indulge in behaviors which expose them to the risk of infection.

At the same time, Sri Lanka has its own internal refugee problem with nearly 300,000 people who have moved out of the north and now live in make-shift refugee camps in central parts of the Island, and a few in Colombo. Some of these women reportedly engage in prostitution as a means of livelihood. And a large majority of their clients are soldiers from the south fighting in the north.

2. POVERTY AND PROSTITUTION

The study indicates that there is no simple link between prostitution and poverty. Poverty is definitely a co-factor and, even in developing countries, it works in combination with social, political, cultural and other factors to abet prostitution. According to IHO, people do not simply look at prostitution as a way out of poverty. However, when a person or family is poor, causes such as rape, incest, broken marriages, and childlessness become critical events. This is more true when formal and informal institutions fail to respond in a supportive and caring manner to such crises.

The *Devdasi* system is a case in point. In India's traditional society, the child dedicated to the temple goddess would have been taken care of by the person who buys the child at the auction. But when children in their thousands are auctioned in this fashion and when adopting families refuse to give them a share of the family inheritance, the ritual becomes a means of initiating them into prostitution .

India affords a further insight into the relationship between poverty and prostitution, particularly in the context of development strategies. A large proportion of its population depends on subsistence fishing or agriculture which are by definition fragile economies. Natural or socio-economic upheavals including mass migration as refugees-for example, the one lakh refugees from Bangladesh in Bombay, and fishing communities displaced by multinationals allowed into prawn culture along the coast of Tamil Nadu—can be devastating.

This is so because traditional mechanisms for coping with poverty fail to operate in the changing context due to its sheer magnitude or suddenness of impact. Thus, it is not surprising that several members of the sex industry in Bombay and Madras come from population groups subjected to such crises. The sudden closure of mills in Ahmedabad is another example of economic disorientation rather than poverty *per se* which is the underlying causal factor. The analogue at the individual level would be a victim of rape, incest or failed marriage.

In the absence of coping mechanisms for both individuals and communities in crisis, organized prostitution, with its network of brokers, procurers, pimps and brothel owners found in all three countries, has been a contributory factor. The rising fear of AIDS, and increasing police repression has also led to more people being brought into the sex industry through such networks. Thus, the individual or community in crisis is the most vulnerable and likely candidate for prostitution.

It is important to note that prostitution is not only proscribed by law in all the four countries, but is actively condemned as an immoral means of earning a livelihood. Thus, for an individual to disregard social mores or the law and take to prostitution, the circumstances must be extremely compelling.

Tragically, however, in most cases the compelling reasons are not absolute poverty. Which means that it is not the lack of basic needs like food, clothing and shelter, but the perception that they are poor compared to others in their society. Specific examples of this tragic situation are Thailand and Malaysia which are being rapidly absorbed into the international consumer culture. Being a simple farmer or a plantation worker is just not enough. One can make much more money from prostitution than from farming !

VIII. ETHICAL ISSUES

The main ethical issue concerning sex workers is testing them for HIV In Malaysia, for instance, once sex workers are taken into police custody and produced before a court of law, testing becomes mandatory. In Thailand, sex workers in brothels are required by the management to undergo quarterly tests and maintain a health card or record. Anonymous unlinked tests are conducted in all countries for surveillance purposes. Most NGOs object to testing of any kind for sex workers. The issue is discussed in relation to the three countries as follows:

INDIA

The GAP Director felt that testing only serves an academic or scientific purpose, disregarding consequences for the individual who is found positive. She also feels that it gives the rest of society a false sense of security originating from the belief that HIV is confined to the so-called "epicenters". At the same time, the procedure targets sex workers as the culprits thereby increasing their social rejection and repression. Police raids, abuse and criminalisation of sex workers has therefore increased along with tests showing high HIV rates among them.

The problem is further complicated by the fact that agencies carrying out testing do not have pre or post-test counselling. And there are no remedial social action or services for those who are found to be positive. IHO states that its counselling services are used by some sex workers from Bombay, but the normal practice among positive sex workers is to move from one location to another to avoid stigmatization by peers or losing their jobs. IHO social workers recall how results which are positive can be psychologically disastrous for the sex worker who is already depressed considering the past experience of exploitation. Testing may also give the sex worker a false sense of security if found negative, making him or her believe that past behaviour patterns with regard to sex are free of risk.

MALAYSIA

Sex workers and drug users are subjected to mandatory testing if taken into police custody. Here again, no counselling services are provided. As a result, criminalisation of sex workers has increased with the advent of HIV. During the research period, the government was planning to set up a rehabilitation-cum-detention center for HIV positive sex workers. Some NGOs who had been approached for help in this matter, showed reluctance, contending that the country's law pertaining to communicable diseases could be used to detain them indefinitely even till their death; a process tantamount to incarceration.

THAILAND

Female sex workers in direct prostitution, meaning brothels, are routinely tested for STD and HIV. Some managers keep track of the examination results in order to maintain that their establishment is free of AIDS. Recalled G.C: "They keep lists and make sure the sex workers go on schedule. Although testing is not mandatory, and confidentiality is maintained by the clinic, the managers have access to the results. If a girl is positive, she is dismissed. The absence of support services for positive sex workers only helps in spreading of the epidemic: They go and join another establishment or, as a last resort, work in the streets."

Where girls are in bondage, even if found positive, they are not allowed to leave the establishment until their debt is paid-. A sex worker's experience in a similar predicament was recounted by ACCESS Director. "The girl from northern Thailand worked in a massage parlour, and her family owed 25,000 bhat to the agent. When she went to have the quarterly test and was found to be positive by the local health authorities she was told that her health card would be seized. But since she wanted to continue working, she pleaded with them. Feeling sorry, they returned her card. Most such sex workers with HIV are still working in the sex industry. This girl came to us for help as she had not been given any counselling."

What then is the entire purpose behind testing of sex workers other than mere compiling of statistics? Is it ethical to test them and leave them without counselling?

IX. SUMMARY OF FINDINGS AND CONCLUSIONS

HIV/AIDS Statistics and NGOs

An observation found common to practically all situations surveyed is the lack of agreement between official (government) statistics and estimates provided by NGOS. The difference in estimates is quite wide and is probably a result of using different sources of data. Particularly interesting is the correlation made by the Indian Health Organization (IHO) between the degree of urbanization and incidence of HIV. While this may be true for Maharashtra (India), in Thailand higher rates of HIV have been reported from peripheral areas in the north.

Sex Workers

Sex workers comprise a relatively large population in urban areas, and even in a city like Bombay their numbers are astronomical. In context of the HIV epidemic it is disconcerting to note that, compared to their numbers, the participation of NGOS is very small. In the course of 10 years IHO, for example, has been able to reach and teach one third of the sex worker population in Bombay's brothels. EMPOWER's efforts for a similar period, on the other hand, has been limited to 3000 out of a total of 200,000 sex workers in Thailand (The latter figure being a minimum, excluding sex workers who are street walkers).

If actual number of sex workers are taken into consideration, NGO activity of the present scale will just not be able to halt the progressing epidemic. The answer lies, not in having more NGOs, but in harnessing their experience and strategies within existing government infrastructure. Most governments, however, appear to have palmed off the task of AIDS prevention among sex workers to NGOs. However, they have done so without even providing adequate financial and institutional support so that the latter could expand their current levels of operation. Unless this impasse is solved, all NGO activity would be reduced to only an interesting academic exercise.

Sex workers happen to be a highly diverse population group representing, even in the same country, different age groups, regions, language groups, and ethnic-religious groups. The complexity in gender terms is also notable. Although female sex workers form a majority, the population also includes a significant number of eunuchs, transvestites, and MSMs (Males who have sex with males). Working with such a complex population has meant using different strategies for building trust and promoting safe sex behaviour. The presence of a large number of 'non-females' adds another dimension to the thesis that transmission of HIV in Asian countries would be mainly through heterosexual means.

Practically all sex workers are socially and psychologically disadvantaged; and at the bottom of the hierarchy are female sex workers. Lack of education, inadequate knowledge of HIV and STD, poor living condition, low wages; and the inability to talk back to clients, law enforcement officers, and exploiters are some of the disabilities arising out of the generally submissive role of women in Asian society. Although unionization and empowerment are *sine qua nons* for protection from HIV, how far this objective will be realized in the short term is not clear.

Sex workers are also a highly mobile group; excepting women working as bonded sex workers in the brothels of Thailand, or those who are supplied to brothels by agents on a contract basis. Geographical mobility is another factor which inhibits taking up programmes and prevents proper monitoring of safe sex initiatives.

Building Trust

A variety of methods have been used to build trust and win the confidence of sex workers. Some preliminary measures include socializing, talking about their daily problems and finding answers and solutions to them. Using kinship terms, like sister or aunt, when addressing them could also be helpful. Similarly affectionately touching them, showing concern, listening, and helping to cope with personal or health crisis such as STDs, reconciliation with families, and counselling (if the sex worker is HIV positive) also helps. Having won over the sex worker's confidence, asking for the sex worker's cooperation in implementing programmes is much easier.

For reaching out to sex workers living under a management or external control, winning the confidence of brothel owners, pimps and managers is important. Giving such people an important role as educators, advisers, and change agents has been one way of mobilizing their support and reducing suspicions about the NGO's intentions. In some situations brothel managers have been persuaded to cooperate by explaining to them that it makes better business sense if the sex workers are in good health. In others, winning the trust of informal leaders among sex workers proved indispensable. Employing social workers who are themselves sex workers and therefore familiar with the local language and circuits is another effective strategy.

Winning trust also depends on personal qualities of the change agent such as persistence, patience and courage. This is important because he or she has to venture virtually into foreign domain, particularly when working among-street walkers. Recruiting people who have such abilities and traits has proved to be difficult, partly due to the strong social stigma attached to both prostitution and HIV/AIDS. This probably explains why the intervention activities have been slow and limited in scope.

Supporting Self-Help Initiatives of Sex Workers

It needs to be stated that sex workers themselves do not take any initiative on their own. Instead, NGOs have to assess their needs and stimulate participation in relevant initiatives. These include improving knowledge of STDs and HIV, and providing non-formal education for sex workers who have left school early or have not had any schooling at all. One also has to motivate them to take up responsibility for the health of other sex workers, promote self-confidence and self-respect through their participation in seminars and workshops. Besides, one needs to provide simple skills such as sewing, language, typing, opening a bank account, learning about civic amenities and resources; skills which may be of help later on in life. It is also important to provide legal education and representation; promotion of self-expression through group counselling, voicing feelings and emotions through talks and writing of articles, participating in dramas, and exploring possibilities of forming unions.

In most such ventures, non-female sex workers were found to be more assertive and responsive, and showed more leadership qualities. Perhaps, some day, movements to unionize or fight for the rights of all sex workers will see non-female sex workers in the vanguard.

Feasibility of Safe Sex

Most NGO personnel believe that 10.0 per cent safe sex is possible. However, conditions needed for making it happen are so many, and so unlikely to be put into practice, that it is just not feasible in the short term. At best, NGOs have been successful in disbursing condoms among sex workers. But that, however, does not ensure their being put to use.

Obstacles in the way of 100 per cent safe sex: (a) lack of literacy and awareness of STD and HIV, (b) language barriers between educators and sex workers, (c) fear of police arrest which detors sex workers from carrying condoms or taking sufficient time to negotiate, (d) lack of unity or unionization, so that sex workers cannot take a stand against customers unwilling to use condoms, (e) reluctance among female sex workers to try alternatives to vaginal sex due to cultural taboos against fondling male genitals or having oral sex, (f) unavailability of good quality condoms, (g) expectations of sex workers that it is the change agent's responsibility to have condoms delivered at their doorstep, (h) social taboos on purchasing condoms from shops or other public outlets, and (i) lack of resources for NGOs to monitor whether condoms distributed have been used.

Almost all these barriers to safe sex will continue to exist for some time to come, if not for ever. Some of them could, of course, change if public attitudes towards sex workers become less intolerant and governments amended laws relating to prostitution. However, given the prevaling attitude, even these simple things happening are a remote possibility. Claims that 100 per cent safe sex has been achieved in certain countries are untenable, considering that monitoring methods adopted by (government) agencies are often intimidatory in nature.

These problems apart, safe sex can be ensured only if the sex worker is convinced about such safe practices; and thereby insists on the customer wearing a condom. They must also have a professional attitude towards sex, clients and towards their workrather than thinking of it as a chore. For drug users the problem gets more complicated, because then the driving force behind commercial sex becomes making money for sustaining the habit. Education about safe sex should, therefore, be made a persistent counselling activity.

Unless sex workers insist on condom use all efforts to empower them will be rendered ineffective. In most situations, refusing to have sex is an option left to the customer and not the sex worker. The possible loss of income, and even the prospect of being physically manhandled by the customer have been the main reasons for this. A major share of the responsibility for safe sex and for spread of HIV has, therefore, to be taken by the clients.

This means the need for a crash programme of intensive public education on safe sex methods throughout the length and breadth of Asia. No NGO has such a capability. Only governments have the resources and manpower to launch educational campaigns of such magnitude; NGOs could, of course, help with their expertise. As a preliminary step, it would be mutually beneficial for the relevant NGOs and government agencies to get together on a common platform and work out modalities of educational and other activities.

Education and empowerment alone are not enough to ensure that safe sex becomes a reality, unless it is also enforced. Imposing a certain behaviour pattern to something as intimate as sex is, however, just not possible, either by a government, any NGO or even by the sex workers themselves.

In this regard, a useful lesson can be learnt from an event that took place in Chaing Kom District in northern Thailand where a Brothel Owners Association decided to force clients to use condoms. Although such a measure could not cover street walkers, it at least provided protection from HIV to a large proportion of sex workers in brothels.

Corridors and Links with Poverty

Highways and truck routes are a principal source of HIV transmission across populations in all the four countries studied, though to a lesser extent in the island country of Sri Lanka. In addition, pilgrimage centers and fairs attract both sex workers and clients. Commuting across national boundaries for cheap sex, and the flow of large number of migrant workers from one country to another are processes which accelerate transmission. Measures for public education on HIV prevention should therefore be carried out not only within countries, but across the region.

Poverty is seen as an important co-factor, rather than the sole cause of growing prostitution. Other factors include personal crisis due to rape, abduction, incest or failed marriages. A community crisis due to economic disorientation brought about by the failure of harvests, civil strife, and displacement of communities as a result of large financial ventures can also lead to prostitution. Failure of supportive institutions to cope with such crises is also a co-factor. Relative—and not absolute—poverty can also push people into prostitution, as a means of making quick money and being part of the new consumerist culture. The emergence of crime syndicates that buy and supply sex workers is yet another development in Asia.

Ethical Issues

Testing sex workers for HIV, without providing adequate counselling, especially for those who are found positive, is another issue of ethical concern. Tests are ordered by a court of law following the arrest of sex workers, or are conducted by brothel owners who wish to maintain a good image of their establishments. Once a sex worker is pronounced positive, unless bonded, she loses employment. The effect of the verdict is also psychologically disastrous.

2

Sharing The Challenge of AIDS Prevention

The Community Aids Service Penang

JENNY HUDDART

NOTES ON USING THE CASE

1. In addition to these notes, the materials relating to the Community AIDS Service Penang organisation consist of:
   (a) Learning Objectives;
   (b) Discussion Questions;
   (c) The Case;
   (d) Facilitators' Notes
2. The discussion questions are intended to help readers to focus on what are considered to be particularly important issues illustrated in the Case. However, the Case may highlight other interesting points and you are encouraged to examine, analyse and discuss these with others.
3. You should review the Objectives and Discussion Questions before turning to the Case itself. After reading the Case carefully, you should then return to the Discussion Questions and prepare your own responses to these, making notes as appropriate, before discussing the case with others.

4. Doing something oneself is the most effective method of learning. Therefore, to get the maximum benefit from the Case, you should prepare your own analysis of the Case before comparing this with points raised in the Facilitators' Notes.
5. There are no right or wrong answers to the Discussion Questions posed. The important issue is the ability to analyse the factors that are influencing the situation and the use of this analysis to draw conclusions about the future.
6. The case is intended to facilitate discussion on important organisational and programmatic issues; it is not intended to demonstrate good or bad practices, nor to evaluate the work of the organisation represented.

Objectives

1. To explore and evaluate the HIV/AIDS prevention role of NGOs in places where cultural or religious beliefs and practices make it difficult to use strategies promoted in less conservative environments .
2. To develop participants' understanding of the organisational issues that may be faced by a volunteer-based NGO as it responds to the needs for HIV/AIDS education and support interventions.
3. To identify the strategies that can be used to maintain the organisational effectiveness of a small, volunteer-based NGO.

Discussion Questions

1. What role did CASP play in Malaysia's response to HIV/AIDS? What were the benefits and possible disadvantages of its approach? What other strategies might CASP have considered?
2. What were the difficulties that faced CASP as an organisation? What suggestions could you make to the new Committee on the strategies and approaches it might use to maintain the viability and cohesion of CASP in the future?
3. What suggestions could you make to the Committee in relation to CASP's future programme activities and funding?
4. What suggestions could you make to the new Committee on how it might prepare its next funding proposal?

MALAYSIA AND HIV/AIDS

The Malaysian peninsula is bordered by Thailand to the North and Singapore to the South. The States of Sabah and Sarawak and the Federal Territory of Labuan are separated from peninsular Malaysia by the South China Sea and border the Indonesian island of Kalimantan. In 1992, Malaysia had a total estimated population of 18 million, made up of approximately 61% Malays, 30% Chinese and 8% Indian. More than 42% of the population fell into the 15-39 year age group. The official religion of Malaysia is Islam, although other religions, particularly Buddhism, Hinduism and Christianity are practiced freely. Bahasa Malaysia is the official language, but English, Tamil and Chinese languages are both widely used and taught in schools and colleges.

In the early 90's, Malaysia's economy was booming but short of labour. A 1990 survey found that the manufacturing sector alone was short of between 50,000 and 80,000 workers, while the Malaysian Agricultural Producers Association stated that plantation output could drop by one third if foreigners were to leave. To fill the gap, thousands of workers were coming to work in Malaysia, both legally and illegally, from Indonesia, Bangladesh, the Philippines and other poorer countries in Asia. Although numbers were probably small, there were frequent articles in the press about migrant sex workers, particularly those from Thailand. More than 3.8 million tourists visited Malaysia in 1991.

Malaysia recognised that it had a serious problem with drug addiction. In 1991, there were reported to be more than 100,000 injecting drug users, most favouring heroin. To control the situation, Malaysia inflicted severe penalties for drug use and had retained the sentence of death for trafficking.

The first AIDS case in Malaysia was detected in December, 1986. A proactive surveillance programme, launched in 1989 to screen injecting drug users in Government correctional centres and medical institutions, resulted in an apparently sharp rise in HIV+ cases around that time. In January 1991, there were 750 officially-reported cases of HIV infection in the country, and 19 people suffering from AIDS. By August 1992, the figure was 3,735 HIV+ persons, while the number of AIDS cases had risen to a total of 60, of whom 40 had died. Of those identified as HIV+, by far the largest proportion were still injecting drug users, although blood donor screening had detected an annual doubling in the incidence rate of HIV infection since 1987.

As reports of AIDS in Asia appeared in the news, Malaysian papers carried articles under headings such as "Killer Disease Found in Malaysia" and "Man Gets AIDS in Hospital through Blood Mix-up". Widespread fear and a lack of clear information resulted in misunderstandings and misapprehensions about HIV transmission.

Blood banks in many hospitals ran dry as donors stayed away for fear of contracting AIDS. Published figures on HIV infection rates among the Thai sex workers led to local newspaper articles and letters condemning promiscuous behaviour and calls for the Government to test all suspected prostitutes for HIV infection, to close down 'vice dens' and to prevent HIV+ foreigners from entering the country. The Ministry of Health, aware of both the facts of HIV transmission and the experiences of other countries in their efforts to stem infection rates, was making efforts to educate the public. The Ministry was also supporting NGOs in their HIV/AIDS efforts, providing such organisations as the Pink Triangle with technical assistance and AIDS education materials. But the argument that 'prevention was more important than human rights' was being forcibly made, and in late 1991, the Ministry was directed by the Cabinet to study various proposals for containing the epidemic. (Exhibit 1.)

THE LAUNCH OF THE COMMUNITY AIDS SERVICE PENANG

During 1989, individuals from the gay community in Penang began to discuss the HIV/AIDS situation in the country. Some already had direct experience of trying to help individuals who were concerned about their HIV status and were seeking blood tests. Others had seen the fear and discrimination faced by those identified as HIV+. Public education at that time was focussed on the need to avoid sexual contact with those from "high-risk groups"; this gave a false sense of security to people outside of those groups, whilst providing little practical information on how to protect against infection to those who did see themselves as being at risk.

In November 1989, CASP was launched with seven founding members, drawn from the University (both Malaysian citizens and expatriate faculty on contract), the Penang Family Planning Association (FPA), and other private sector organisations. All were volunteers to CASP, holding full-time jobs elsewhere. The group agreed on its aims and objectives (Exhibit 2), and submitted their constitution for formal registration with the Registrar of Societies. Until registration was formally granted, an organisation could not conduct fund-raising activities or receive external funding. By early 1992, the application to register CASP with the Registrar of Societies had been approved. Once registered, CASP would have to submit annual reports to the Registrar of Societies including the minutes of its Committee meetings, the total number of paid-up members, and audited financial statements.

THE FIRST THREE YEARS

AIDS Education for the General Public

CASP's first HIV/AIDS education activities were carried out in conjunction with the Penang FPA in various factories, schools and youth groups. CASP members also provided a ready entry to the university for AIDS prevention talks to both staff and students.

November 1989 also saw the beginning of CASP's collaboration with the Pink Triangle Malaysia when the latter visited Penang to provide an educational show at a local nightclub. 1989 was also the first year that CASP participated in World AIDS Day activities; for the 1991 World AIDS Day CASP set up a stall at the Penang ferry terminal, selling books on AIDS, CASP key rings and T-shirts; giving out free pamphlets. Where CASP has seen the need, it has produced its own information materials, including posters, leaflets and instructions on proper condom use. To offset some of its costs and as a means of advertising CASP services, key-rings, pens and T-shirts have been printed and sold.

Advocacy for Effective National Prevention Policies

In Malaysia, 'Letters to the Editor' of the newspapers have traditionally been a way of conducting public debate of important issues. CASP used this medium to full advantage, despite the fact that this might antagonise those of differing views. When news of the Cabinet's directive to the Ministry of Health appeared in the papers (Exhibit 1), CASP responded rapidly, taking the opportunity to present the experience of other countries and the negative consequences of discriminating against those infected with HIV (Exhibit 3).

Hotline for AIDS Information and Counselling

In March and April 1990, Pink Triangle Malaysia provided Hotline Counselling training for CASP members and a few student volunteers from the university. By October of that year, a telephone had been installed in the home of one of the members and a roster of members and volunteers drawn up to man the hotline from 7:30 pm to 9:30 pm every Tuesday and Thursday. Some members already had previous counselling experience, and at the start of the hotline service, a newly-trained counsellor would be paired with someone more experienced. CASP was careful to restrict the extent of the Hotline service to a level that it felt it could consistently maintain.

Advertisements for the Hotline were placed in the local newspaper, but frequently they were withdrawn by the newspaper after the first appearance. Subsequently, as CASP began to produce its own HIV/AIDS information materials, it always included details of the hotline service and number. Hotline details were also given out at all of CASP's AIDS education talks and events. Calls to the hotline tended to increase whenever news about HIV/AIDS was prominent in the media; during quiet times, few if any calls were received. Most of the calls have heen to ask for factual information about HIV/AIDS; a few callers have discussed their personal concerns. Two further training sessions on telephone counselling were held in 1991. Before the second programme, CASP placed an advertisement in the paper calling for volunteers to attend the training and to help man the hotline. Several people did apply and joined the training, but very few of them subsequently became active volunteers.

Pre and Post HIV Test Counselling

In early 1991, building on the Hotline training, CASP members decided to offer counselling for those who were considering taking an HIV test, to refer them to a private laboratory for confidential testing, to accompany them to the test, and to offer further counselling at the time of the test result. Up to August 1992, although some individuals had made the decision to seek an HIV test, few had actually turned up for their appointment at the laboratory. CASP was also concerned that it had not yet been able to identify a suitably trained and sympathetic doctor to whom individuals who tested HIV positive could be referred for any necessary treatment.

AIDS Education for Hotel Staff

In 1991, one CASP member whose husband provided her with access to the Penang Hoteliers' Association, was able to discuss the implications of HIV infection at one of the Association's meetings. Afterwards, she made contact with individual hotel managers and one of these agreed to allow CASP to talk to their managers and staff. Hearing of the success of this first talk, other hotel managers then requested CASP's help, and by the end of 1991, CASP had visited each of the major hotels in Penang. These hotels had a very high staff turnover; CASP was aware that AIDS education talks would have to be repeated frequently, but a shortage of experienced members was a problem in sustaining this programme. CASP was also instrumental in persuading the hotels to install condom vending machines in both the gents and the ladies washrooms. This was a major step since, until that time, condoms could only be obtained through private pharmacies or, if the client was married, through the family planning programme at Government and FPA facilities.

The hotel staff education programme led to another opportunity for CASP, this time to reach young people through the hotel discotheques. CASP members used their own children to help them recruit a number of youngsters willing to talk to their peers. CASP provided them with information about HIV transmission and prevention and then accompanied them into the discos where they shared this information and distributed leaflets and condoms.

Sex Worker Outreach Programme

In August 1992, CASP had just started an outreach programme for sex workers on the streets of Penang. Once a week, a small team of members would visit the working area of the female prostitutes and transvestites and would distribute leaflets and free condoms to both the sex workers and their clients. The sex workers and the CASP members were gradually building recognition and trust, which CASP hoped would lead to more open information exchange and permit the development of other support programmes for this group.

CASP AS AN ORGANISATION

By August 1992, only one of the founding members was still with CASP. Some had moved away from Penang, some had found that the demands on their time had become excessive, some had become uncomfortable with CASPis working style and choice of activities.

However, new individuals had filled their places and CASP had a total of 50 individuals on their mailing list, of whom 20 were paid-up and active members. The recent annual members' meeting had elected a new nine-member Committee and the appointees were busy considering strategies for the future.

The amount of work, both programme and administrative, was large for a small group of volunteers to deal with in the evenings and weekends. Experience had shown that excessive demands could lead to frustration and tension among members. The CASP Committee knew that they needed to increase the number of active members, but previous drives to do so had not had the expected results.

In addition, few of the newly-recruited volunteers had contributed to the extent anticipated. Some had been unable to give much time to the work of CASP; others simply drifted away from the group. It was sometimes difficult to integrate new members into the organisation, especially since most had little or no previous experience of HIV/AIDS education or counselling. By August 1992, CASP members were wondering whether enough effort had been made in the past to make these new volunteers feel useful from the very beginning and were considering what strategies they might use in the future to attract and retain new members.

Another issue being considered by the Committee was how to reconcile the different interests, needs and priorities of the members. CASP volunteers came from a wide variety of backgrounds and brought different skills and ideas to the group. There were differences in working style: some preferred to work as a loosely knit group, without a clearly defined hierarchy; others were accustomed to and felt more comfortable with a more formal working environment. Views on the approach that CASP should take also varied: some members felt that CASP should be a 'pathfinder', taking an independent and sometimes aggressive role in promoting effective HIV prevention; others felt that CASP should take a more cautious approach and work more closely with, or under the umbrella of, official agencies.

In July and August 1990, two CASP members had attended an AIDS conference in Australia during which it was suggested that CASP apply for financial support from the Australian International Development Aid Bureau (AIDAB). As a result, CASP submitted a proposal to AIDAB which resulted in a 12-month commitment of A$12,500 for the establishment of the Hotline, covering telephone equipment, office and telephone costs, counselling training, and the purchase of audio-visual equipment for AIDS education. Advance funding for the first quarter eventually arrived in August, 1991; subsequent quarterly funding was to be released following receipt of a progress report and financial statement from CASP.

In January 1992, CASP had felt it necessary to move its operations out of members' homes into a proper office and had managed to find a landlord willing to rent to them. But the rental and utility costs represented a significant monthly outlay. To add further financial pressure, by August 1992, the final quarters' funds from AIDAB had not yet been released since CASP's progress report and accounts for the previous three months were still outstanding.

During 1991, CASP had developed and submitted a second funding proposal to AIDAB, this time covering a three-year period. This proposal included continued funding for CASP's existing activities, together with several new initiatives. (See Exhibit 4.) By August 1992, although the first project funding period was officially over, no response had yet been received from AIDAB in relation to a second phase of funding. CASP's new Committee had much to think about.

EXHIBIT 1

The New Straits Times, 19 September, 1991

MINISTRY TOLD TO STUDY AIDS SETTLEMENT

BY ALEX CHOONG

KUALA LUMPUR, Wed. The Cabinet has directed the Health Ministry to study the possiblility of establishing a "settlement" for those suffering from Acquired Immune Definciency Syndrome (AIDS).

This is aimed at confining AIDS patients to a particular place, similar to many leprosy victims who are living at the Sugei Buloh Leprosy Control Centre.

Health Minister Datuk Lee Kim Sai said this was among five proposals which the Cabinet today instructed the Ministry to study.

It is believed that Cuba is the only country so far to have set up a "settlement" for AIDS victims.

Besides having the "settlement", Cuba has also made it complsory for citizens to undergo blood tests.

Other proposals to check the spread of the killer disease are to:

* Study the possibility of imposing the most severe punishment-caning and a jail termon those involved in bringing in foreign prostitutes suffering from AIDS;
* Study how to protect the public from people suffering from AIDS (at the moment it is difficult to differentiate a person suffering from AIDS from those not afflicted with the deadly disease);
* Identify people suffering from AIDS and ensure that they are issued with a special card; and,
* Have provisions under the Infectious Diseases Act to disclose the identity of an AIDS victim.

Private doctors are required to inform the Ministry of notificable diseases listed under the Act.

On the reactions of people suffering from AIDS, Datuk Lee categorised them under three groups.

The first is normally shocked to learn that they are suffering from AIDS while the second feels regretful and remorseful.

The third group, he added, would not be shocked because they knew the consequences of being an AIDS carrier.

Meanwhile, a Ministry source said statistics made available on the AIDS situation in Thailand showed that for every three prostitutes in Bangkok, one is an AIDS victim.

"In Chiengmai it is 4 to 1 and in Haadyai 5 to 1," the source added.

EXHIBIT 2

Aims and Objectives

Cognizant that the problem of AIDS (Acquired Immune Deficiency Syndrome) is a global concern and that Malaysia is not spared from the spread of the disease, we have formed the Community AIDS Service Penang. This project will carry out the following aims and objectives without prejudice towards any individual or group regardless of race, creed, social behaviour, sexuality or nationality.

1. To provide information of AIDS and AIDS prevention to the public.
2. To promote the awareness and practice of safer sex.
3. To encourage changes of behaviours and habits which are likely to lead to HIV (Human Immune Deficiency Virus) infection.
4. To facilitate confidential AIDS testing services.
5. To provide confidential and free counselling on AIDS and on AIDS-related issues, including AIDS test follow-up counselling.
6. To provide telephone counselling services.
7. To devise specific information and education strategies on AIDS prevention related to high-risk behaviours.
8. To cooperate with the Malaysian Government, National and international organisation.
9. To promote Malaysian strategies on AIDS to be fully consonant with international efforts.
10. To work against the stigmatisation and discrimination of persons with AIDS (PWAs)and persons living and/or associated with them.
11. To uphold the rights of PWAs to employment, housing, insurance and all other basic human rights.
12. To promote the availability of and access to necessary medical service for PWAs.
13. To facilitate shelter and other forms of support services for PWAs.
14. To recruit and train volunteers for the organisation.
15. To raise funds through grants and donations and other fund-raising activities for the purpose of carrying out the above aims objectives.

AIDS test proposal not a wise move

UNTIL recently international and local professionals and volunteers working on AIDS have been impressed by the rational approach that the Health Ministry has taken towards the AIDS epidemic, an approach which has closely tracked the policy guidelines of the World Health Organisatmn.

The proposed amendment to the Medical Act 1971 and the Prevention and Control of Infectious Diseases Act, 1988, is the first severe deviation from that policy.

Such a policy shift is antithetical to effective AIDS prevention in Malaysia.

Besides being a dangerous infringement of the basic right of the individual to privacy and authority over his/her own body, the amendment, as it is described in the press, also reflects little understanding of the dynamics of this epidemic and will only help the disease to spread by hampering government and non-government AIDS education programmes.

A climate of fear has been created by the press statements about the amendment.

People whom we are trying to reach with our education programmes now have justifiable fear that their participation may lead to government surveillance of their bodily fluids and their lives.

The number of calls coming into our hotline has suddenly dropped since announcement of the proposed amendment began appearing in the press several weeks ago.

We are reminded of Dr. Jonathan Mann, former director of WHO's Global Programme on AIDS, who warned in an interview in the International AIDS Conference Bulletin in March 1989:

If you have good education and services but the general social climate Is discriminatory and stigmatising, then prevention just won't work.

The Health Ministry's argument for implementing the amendment is based on invalid and unrealistic assumptions:

- THE ministry argues that coercive screening of targeted groups is for the good of the society and that human nights must be balanced against the need to prevent the spread of AIDS .

Actually, the issue of Public Health vs Individual Rights has no place in the reality of AIDS Prevention and Control.

Education programmes are recognised by AIDS professionals throughout the world as the only effective AIDS prevention strategy.

But education programmes work only in an atmosphere free from legal repression and stigmatisation, as reiterated in 1990 by Dr. Daniel Tarantola, Chief of National Programme Support, WHO's Global Programme on AIDS:

* "Education is the key to AIDS prevention;
* Public health must be safeguarded and in order to achieve this, human rights must be protected"

For AIDS education to be effective there must be a willing public that can ask questions and learn to protect themselves without fear of recrimination or discrimination.

In an atmosphere of legal suppression, AIDS prevention measures, no matter how extensive or intensive, will not be effective, and the public health will, decline.

This is supported by the findings of the WHO Australian Inter-Regional Ministerial Meeting on AIDS, 1987, attended by Malaysia's then Health Minister:

* FAR from leading to cure or treatment, the danger of widespread mandatory testing for AIDS is that it will lead on to discrimination, . . . whilst at the same time entirely failing effectively to protect the general community.
* ATTEMPTS to rely upon the criminal law (for AIDS prevention) tend to produce the corruption of public officials; the growth of underground activities; the sense of persecution and oppression in those subject to such laws; . . . and a lack of respect for the law in groups in the community.

The same conclusion regarding the need to protect human rights in public health policy planning and implementation was reached by the 148 national delegates at World Summit of Ministers of Health on programmes for AIDS.

Furthermore, the "Report of the WHO Meeting on Criteria for HIV Screening Programmes" (1987) concluded that mandatory HIV Testing was ineffectual in controlling AIDS:

** READILY accessible counselling and testing for antibody to HIV, provided on a voluntary basis, are more likely to result in behavioural changes that contribute to reducing the spread of HIV than are mandatory screening unitia*tives.

A tested individual is still not an educated individual. Once a person is fully educated in safe sex and AIDS prevention, testing becomes irrelevant.

AIDS prevention is possible only if everyone is taught how to practise prevention, not just those who are HIV positive or in so-called "high risk groups."

When it comes to AIDS, everyone is at risk. Most AIDS professionals threw out the term "high risk group" five years as a distortion of the facts. Why is this inaccurate and discriminatory jargon still being used to justify a controversial law in Malaysia?

Furthermore, if the ministry insists on using the term "high risk group" under this proposed amendment, then heterosexual men and women must be proclaimed the "highest risk group" in Malaysia worldwide.

Since at least 90 per cent of drug addicts, prostitutes, and those infected by transfused blood products are heterosexual and engage in heterosexual sex, over 95 per cent of those presently identified as HIV positive in Malaysia are heterosexual. Obviously this means that everyone is at risk of being infected. AIDS does not discriminate, so why should we?

The proposed amendment:

* WILL break the trust between the Health Ministry and the Malaysian public, creating an atmosphere rife with subterfuge and suspicion. We believe that the less the Health Ministry associates itself with legal actions or social control measures, the more effective it will be in educating the public.
* WILL stigmatise a large body of Malaysian citizens and make these people suspicious of effons to educate and change risky behaviours. It will also lull those not in the so-called "high-risk groups" particularly young people into false security, making them more resistant to education as well.
* WILL handicap the Government's ability to carry out epidemiological studies, because the voluntary data that such studies rely upon will not be forth coming in a climate of repression and because, when HIV is identified in any one population group, it has already spread beyond that group (1990, Dr. Michael Mershon, Director of the WHO Global Programme on AIDS).
* WILL undercut the bona fide out-reach and education programmes of the NGOs and the ministry.
* WILL contravene the Health Ministry's own stated policy of providing pre-test/ post-test counselling to every person tested, because of sheer numbers and because counselling is only possible in a non-coercive situation. The ministry is in danger of making a mockery of its own stated policies and guidelines.
* IGNORES the fact that antibody testing is effective only three months or more following infection, hence each individual would have to be tested every three months for the rest of their lives for an accurate appraisal. Furthermore the test is invalidated, if, five minutes after the blood sample is taken, the subject is exposed to the virus.
* WILL waste valuable resources on coercive testing, diverting desperately needed funds and energies away from education and counselling programmes.

* WILL isolate Malaysia from the community of nations and organisations working together to combat AIDS while preserving individual and cultural rights.

The above negative implications and consequences for Malaysian citizens and the Malaysian public health system, force us to respectfully urge the Health Ministry to withdraw the proposed amendment to the Prevention and Control of Infectious Diseases Act, 1988.

COMMUNITY AIDS SERVICE, Penang.

Exhibit 4
CASP PROPOSAL FOR AIDAB FUNDING

Activity	*91/92 Funds (MS0000)*	*Proposed Funding (MS)*		
		Yr. 1	*Yr. 2*	*Yr. 3*
1. ON-GOING ACTIVITIES				
A. Office and Hotline Maintenanee				
- Office Rental	5.40			
- Two hotlines	1.08			
- Utilities	1.14			
- Security costs	0.40			
- Equipment & supplies	6.75			
B. Public Education Programme & Outreach				
- Prevention talks with video displays				
- Distribution of condoms	1.50			
- Distribution of CASP printed handouts	1.83			
- Sale of books/key-chains	1.10			
C. HIV Testing Proaramme				
- Pre and post-test counselling				
- Distribution of Safe-Sex & Safe IVDU info.	2.1			
- ELISA and Western Blot test fees				
D. Staff Education and Traininz Programme				
- Telephone counselling trainings (1/yr)	1.5			
- Pre-/post-test counselling training (1/yr)	1.5			
- HIV support counselling training	1.5			
E. Special Events				
- World AIDS Day				
- AIDS Memorial Day (Years 2/3)				
- Conference of Malaysian AIDS NGOs				
Sub-Total	25 ,800	28 ,380		

{Cont.}....			
II. NEW PROGRAMMES			
A. Office & Staff			
- Programme Manager[2]		18,000	
- Resource Library[3]		2,000	
- Volunteer recruitment/promotion[4]		2,000	
- Volunteer per diem (@ M$10/day)		2,000	
Suh-Total		24.000	
B. Sex Worker Outreach			
- Sex-Worker Outreach Education/Peer Group Sponsorship		1.00	
- Education materials/publicity		3.00	
- HIV & syphilis test costs[5]		4.50	
Sub-Total		8.50	
C. HIV + Support Services[6]			
- Publicity & media promotion[7]		2.00	
- Needs assessment & development		1.00	
- Education & counselling[8]		1.00	
- Peer Group Sponshorship		1.00	
Sub-Total		5.00	
D. IVDU Outreach			
- Initiate IVDU Outreach Education			
- Education materials			
- HIV test costs			
- Peer Group Sponsorship			
- Safe sex/IVDU cleaning kits			
Sub-Total			
E. CASP Newsletter			
- Publish on regular basis			
Total	65.88	74.00[9]	85,000[10]

1. Calculated on the basis of +10% over 1991 costs.
2. Qualified programme manager to be hired to carry out the programme approved by the Committee, to oversee all CASP volunteers and administer all CASP programmes and activities.
3. Resource library to include tapes, books, information, posters, prevention and treatment information, epidemiology, politics and legal issues.
4. Includes bringing in experts for volunteer workshops/information updates; hosting a Crisis Intervention workshop for CASP volunteers and staff, etc.
5. Includes Elisa and TPHA (for syphilis) tests at M&30 x 100; and Western Blot Tests at M&150 x 10.
6. Development of support services for people infected with HIV, their families and lovers.
7. Includes advertising on public transport, in cinemas, television, radio and the press, etc.
8. Education programmes on care and treatment of HIV infection and AIDS
9. Increase of 15% on Year 1 programme costs plus costs of new IVDU outreach programme and CASP newsletter. IVDU programme (with similar components to the HIV+ outreach costs in Year 1).
10. Increase on Year 2 costs of 15% to expand all existing programmes.

EXHIBIT 5
1992/93 GRANT REQUEST: PROJECT COST SCHEDULE FOR YEAR 1

OBJECTIVES/OUTPUT	1ST QUARTER			2ND QUARTER			3RD QUARTER			4TH QUARTER			SUB TOTAL (M$000)
	1	2	3	4	5	6	7	8	9	10	11	12	
EXISTING PROGRAMMES Hotline, outreach, public meetings, staff training, new equipment (fax/answering m/c. computer peripherals, software).	7.09			7.09			7.09			7.09			28.38
NEW PROGRAMMES 1. OFFICE AND STAFF:													
Programme manager (mthly wage)	1.50	1.50	1.50	1.50	1.50	1.50	1.50	1.50	1.50	1.50	1.50	1.50	18.00
Resource Library	0.50			0.50			0.50			0.50			2.00
Volunteer Recruit/Promotion	0.50			0.50			0.50			0.50			2.00
Volunteer per diem	0.50			0.50			0.50			0.50			2.00
2. SEX WORKER OUTREACH:													
Ed.& Couns.& Peer Group Support	0.25		0.25	0.25			0.25						1.00
Educ. materials & publicity	2.25			0.25			0.25			0.25			3.00
HIV/Syphilis tests	1.13			1.12			1.13			1.12			4.50
3. HIV+ SUPPORT SERVICES													
Publicity & Media Promotion	0.50			0.50			0.50			0.50			2.00
Needs Assess't & Development	0.25			0.25			0.25			0.25			1.00
Education and Counselling	0.25			0.25			0.25			0.25			1.00
Peer Group Sponsorship	0.25			0.25			0.25			0.25			1.00
TOTAL													65.88

FACILITATORS' NOTES

General Points About Using The Case

1. Participants should be encouraged to read the case and to prepare their own analysis before it is discussed with others in the classroom. The discussion questions should be handed out with thecase to assist participants in their analysis.
2. Generally, discussion of this case has required 1½ to 2 hours (assuming that participants have previously read the case and prepared their own analysis).
3. The discussion questions included with this case are intended to help participants to focus on what were considered to be particularly important issues illustrated in the case. However, the case may highlight many other interesting points for participants and they should be encouraged to examine, analyse and discuss these if raised.
4. The notes that follow are intended to assist the facilitator to prepare to teach the case. They provide a synopsis of the information given in the case, together with some ideas on strategies that CASP might adopt in the future. These notes should not replace the facilitator's own preparation and analysis. At all times, the facilitator should encourage the participants to reach their own conclusions, based upon a thorough analysis of the information given.
5. When introducing participants to the case, the facilitator should stress that the case is intended to facilitate discussion on important organisational and programmatic issues; it is not intended to demonstrate good or bad practices, nor to evaluate the work of CASP.

CASE SYNOPSIS

Discussion Question 1:

What role did CASP play in Malaysia's response to HIV/AIDS? What were the benefits and possible disadvantages of its approach? What other strategies might CASP have considered ?

(a) The role that CASP played:

- Advocacy for protection of the individual's rights and for effective education of the public about HIV/AIDS and ways of protecting themselves. By being willing to speak out (such as through the newspapers) about counter-productive policies and actions, CASP encouraged public debate of the issues.

- CASP's article (Exhibit 3) is based upon facts rather than emotion and draws heavily upon the experiences of other countries as well as quoting from recognised authorities such as WHO and the Malaysian Government itself. By doing this, CASP provided the Government itself with well-founded arguments which it could use in its debate with various interest groups in the country.
- As an NGO, CASP was able to respond more flexibly to HIV/AIDS education needs than the Government services.
- CASP could also gain access to members of the community which Government services could not easily reach.
- CASP's association with the Penang FPA was extremely important in providing CASP with initial access to work sites and youth groups and in providing CASP with a link to a wellestablished and respected NGO.

(b) The benefits and possible disadvantages of CASP's approach:

Benefits

- CASP's independence from the Government health and social service agencies allowed them access to those sections of the community whose activities put them at considerable risk of infection but who would be reluctant to come forward to government officials.
- CASP's independence also allowed them to speak out and carry out activities which would never have been possible if the organisation had formal links with the authorities.
- CASP's willingness to air its views and arguments provided a focus for other like-minded individuals in the community and should have attracted new members who were willing to speak openly about sex and sexuality and how individuals could protect themselves from infection.

Possible Disadvantages

- CASP would have had to exercise some caution to ensure that its activities remained within the limits of tolerance of the authorities. CASP needed to achieve a fine balance between remaining visibly independent of government yet retaining sufficient linkages and mutual respect to be allowed to continue providing services to the general public and those 'on the fringe' of Penang society.

- CASP's outspokenness could lead to some personal difficulties for the Malaysian members. The expatriate members could perhaps afford to take more risks.
- CASP's radical reputation could scare off some potential new members, who might feel more ccmfortable with a more conservative approach. Some of the original members of CASP had left the organisation over this issue.
- CASP had not tried to collaborate with the Ministry of Health or to seek its views on CASP's activities. This could affect CASP's future funding situation in the sense that some sources of external funding for NGOs are channelled through the Government (through NGO Boards or Councils) and CASP might not rank high on a list of NGO's being considered for support.

(c) Other Possible Strategies:

- CASP might have tried to approach those officers in the Ministry of Health responsible for health education to identify whether there was any potential for collaboration on the design or dissemination of HIV/AIDS education materials.
- CASP had ready access to the University faculty and students. Perhaps the University could have been encouraged to mount a regional seminar on a topic such as the social implications of HIV/AIDS and to publish the proceedings as another means of providing influential support for more effective HIV/AIDS education and services.
- CASP could have tried to identify other voluntary groups or NGOs providing social services in Penang and investigated the possibility of collaboration. If feasible, this might help CASP to share its workload as well as to expand the HIV/AIDS education network.

Discussion Question 2:

What were the difficulties that faced CASP as an organisation? What suggestions could you make to the new Committee on the strategies and approaches it might use to maintain the viability and cohesion of CASP in the future?

(a) Difficulties

Implementation problems:

- The length of time taken to register CASP with the Registrar of Societies so that it can offlcially operate as an organisation and receive funding for its activities.

- Some passive opposition to the activities of CASP, such as the difficulties of placing the advertisements for the hotline in the papers.
- A lack of time/stat resources to tollow through on some programs, such as: the need to identify a doctor to treat those identified as HIV+ and the need to follow up with the hotel staff AIDS education programme.
- The general lack of response to the Hotline service, perhaps indicating that CASP members had decided that this was an important service before any significant indications that such a service was needed by the community.

Membership problems:

- Moving from the founding group of friends to a more heterogenous group of members.
- Difficulties in attracting, utilising and retaining new volunteer members.
- Inadequate attention paid to making sure that new members feel that they can make a useful contribution.

Organisational Problems:

- The growing administrative load, even though CASP had only one source of funding. A particularly important problem was that CASP had failed to submit its final quarterly report to AIDAB, thus jeopardising the reimbursement of past expenditures and agreement to a second period of funding.
- The difficulty of reconciling differing interests and views of the members.
- Funding uncertainties, combined with increasing costs related to the office rental, and administrative and programme costs.

(b) Possible Future Strategies

Planning and Implementation:

- Restrict new activities to those that can be sustained by the level and skills of the existing membership .
- Careful identification of priorities for new activities/programs in relation to the needs of the communities to be served and the inputs of other organisations/agencies.

- Monitoring of the progress/success of programme activities to ensure that necessary follow-up to sustain the benefits are included in workplans and funding proposals.

Membership:

- Give each existing member responsibility for identifying potential new members, for briefing them on CASP's aims and activities, and for "looking after them" during the early stages of their membership.
- Development of a simple "induction" programme for potential new members to ensure that each potential recruit is fully aware of CASP's mission (using the mission statement already developed), has the chance to observe CASP's activities, and is encouraged to define for themselves what they believe they can contribute to the organisation before they are accepted as members.
- Ensuring that a specific role is identified and agreed with each new member. Depending on the interests of the individual and on the amount of time that she/he feels able to contribute, a new member might be allocated to work on a specific CASP programme, or to assist in the office (on report production, proposal development, financial accounts, etc.), or to help to identify potential funding sources.
- To try to avoid an overload on the volunteers, CASP needs to control the amount of work it takes on to a level that is reasonable for the number of active members.
- Volunteers need to enjoy their work if they are to continue to contribute willingly and enthusiastically. This can be encouraged by ensuring that members work on areas that interest them, have a specific role and responsibilities, their contribution is recognised, and that there is adequate time for the members to relax and talk about what they are doing.

Organisation:

- Under the umbrella of the main Committee, CASP might organise itself into groups or programmes such that individual programme and managerial interests might be accommodated. This might also help in attracting and retaining new members (see Question 2 above).
- One individual on the Committee might be given specific responsibility for building-'team spirit' and attending to members' concerns. Practical steps that could be taken include:

ensuring that all members are kept informed of what is going on; ensuring that individual's ideas are shared and discussed; making sure that worries are promptly dealt with and allowing concerns relating to the work or the functioning of the organisation to be aired and discussed when necessary; ensuring that no one member becomes over-burdened with work; helping new members to be integrated into the team.

- Allocating specific responsibility for report production, proposal development, financial accounts, etc. to different individuals who have expressed some interest and aptitude for these areas. In particular, ensuring that one person has responsibility for monitoring the funding situation and making sure that the question of future funding remains on the agenda.
- If activities, funding and membership grow, CASP might consider the recruitment of full-time officers. (The second AIDAB proposal includes the salary of a full-time Executive Director).

Discussion Question 3:

What suggestions could you make to the Committee in relation to CASP 'sfuture programme activities and funding ?

(a) Future Programme Activities:

- CASP should be careful not to initiate more activities than it can sustain. By failing to follow up its initial activities with the hotels, for example, CASP might damage its reputation, lose valuable opportunities to provide AIDS education to the hotel staff, forego other possible chances to gain the hotel managers' support for other innovative AIDS prevention activities, and cut off a potential source of financial support.
- There is little indication in the case that CASP has attempted to identify where the largest potential need for HIV/AIDS eclucation and services might lie. CASP might try to approach health and social service organisations on Penang Island to discuss their views, their current activities and their plans. This might help CASP to establish priorities among the long list of possible programmes that they wish to initiate.
- The case states that Malaysia has a large population of migrant workers, both legal and illegal. The probable living conditions and lifestyles of this group would indicate the need fo education on HIV/AIDS and prevention measures. CASP might approach the relevant organisations and government bodies to identify any plans to reach the migrand workers ant to establish whether any sources of funding are available to support such work.

- CASP had already started to develop contact with the Penang sex workers and to gain their trust and cooperation. It might be a good idea if CASP could build on this beginning to identify, with the sex workers, other steps that could be taken to promote condom use, to maintain the general health of the sex workers, or to provide other support and assistance.

(b) Strategies for developing future financial support:

- Allocation of responsibility to one member to ensure that funding issues remain on the agenda at all times.
- More attention to financial accounting (and the necessary progress reports) to ensure that the conditions attached to existing sources of funding are complied with.
- Identification of donors interested in supporting NGO HIV/AIDS programmes.
- Submission of funding proposals to more than one potential funding source, sufficiently in advance of the time funding is required to try to ensure continuity of financing.
- Attempts to develop local sources of programme financing so as to avoid some of the uncertainties, delays conditions and administrative burdens associated with external funding sources. Possible sources might include: (i) charging for the education talks to the hotel staff expanding their HIV/AIDS education activities within the private manufacturing/business sector and establishing a charge for their services; approaching the business sector for contributions in kind to support CASP's activities, such as the printing of T-Shirts, key-rings etc. or the printing and duplicaiton of HIV/AIDS educational materials, the provision of office accommodation, etc.; if permitted, CASP might review the possibility of selling condoms at subsidised rates to the street vendors in the area where the sex workers operate.

Discussion Question 4:

If you were the agency which received CASP's funding proposal, what further information would you request from CASP and why ? What suggestions could you make to the new Committee on how it might prepare its next finding proposal ?

(a) Further Information that might be requested:

- What sort of organisation is CASP? How many staff and volunteers does it have? When was CASP established? Does CASP have a proper accounting system? Is CASP registered as an NGO?

- What previous experience has CASP had in project implementation? What other sources of financial income does CASP have? How will the proposed activities be continued after the project funding ceases?
- What specific activities does CASP intend to implement under this proposed project? Are these activities justified and why?
- How were the budget costs calculated? How much money will be allocated to each activity or item?
- How will the project activities be monitored? What plans does CASP have for evaluating the effectiveness of the activities?

(b) Suggestions for the next funding proposal:

- If the funding agency had no previous dealings with CASP, then the proposal should contain details of the organisation, including its staffing, its experience and its previous and current programmes. In addition, details of previous funding agencies and the achievements of its programmes should be given. This information helps to convince the funding agency that it is dealing with a bona fide and experienced organisation.
- Other sources of support to CASP should be detailed, including member contributions in cash and in-kind, fund raising activities, donations from local sources, etc. This helps to show the potential funder that the NGO's activities and existence would not be entirely reliant on its support.
- Details of how the project was conceived, including background information that led the organisation to design the project and details of what other organisations (if any) are doing to help the problem.
- A description of the aims and objectives of the project and the detailed activities that will be carried out, by whom and when. This is essential for the funding agency to understand the proposal and to evaluate its likelihood of success. A donor cannot be expected to provide support unless it knows the details of how the funds are going to be used.
- An explanation of how the project activities might be continued after the end of the funding period. Funding agencies are often unwilling to initiate a project which appears to represent a long-term commitment on their part.
- A detailed budget tor the project including: unit prices where applicable; a breakdown of the costs for each component activity or item to be procured; a breakdown by year for each line item:

and details of any foreign currency items required (such as imported items, foreign consultants, etc.) If inflation is included in the costs, the level of the increment assumed. This helps the funding agency to confirm that the funding requirements have been carefully planned, that the items and activities to be funded meet their own internal regulations and controls, and provides a base against which project expenditures can subsequently be monitored .

- The proposal budget should include sutticient detail for the funding agency to identify the proposed cash flow as this relates to the proposed activities.

- The proposal should include details of how CASP intends to monitor and evaluate the effectiveness of the proposed activities and programmes. This might forestall the funding agency from imposing its own monitoring and evaluation protocols and would also help the applicant itself to build in adequate time and support for these important activities.

3

Family Planning and AIDS Prevention

The Planned Parenthood Association of Thailand (PPAT)

JENNY HUDDART
MONTU PEKANAN

NOTES ON USING THE CASE

1. In addition to these notes, the materials relating to the Planned Parenthood Association of Thailand consist of:
   (a) Learning Objectives;
   (b) Discussion Questions;
   (c) The Case;
   (d) Facilitators' Notess
2. The discussion questions are intended to help readers to focus on what are considered to be particularly important issues illustrated in the Case. However, the Case may highlight other interesting points and you are encouraged to examine, analyse and discuss these with others.
3. You should review the Objectives and Discussion Questions before turning to the Case itself. After reading the Case carefully, you should then return to the Discussion Questions and prepare your own responses to these, making notes as appropriate, before discussing the case with others.

4. Doing something oneself is the most effective method of learning. Therefore, to get the maximum bepefit from the Case, you should prepare your own analysis of the Case before comparing this with points raised in the Facilitators' Notes.
5. There are no right or wrong answers to the Discussion Questions posed. The important issue is the ability to analyse the factors that are influencing the situation and the use of this analysis to draw conclusions about the future.
6. The case is intended to facilitate discussion on important organisational and programmatic issues; it is not intended to demonstrate good or bad practices, nor to evaluate the work of the organisation represented.

Objectives

1. To explore the benefits and the possible difficulties of integrating family planning and HIV/AIDS prevention programmes and to identify and evaluate strategies that family planning organisations can use to minimise the problems they may face in achieving effective integration.
2. To assess the factors involved in designing, implementing and evaluating effective HIV/AIDS education interventions.
3. To identify and evaluate the management strategies that facilitate an NGO's ability to deal with change and to maintain and develop the effectiveness of its programmes.

Discussion Questions

1. What factors facilitated the addition of HIV/AIDS interventions to PPAT's family planning programmes? What additional factors might influence the integration of HIV/AIDS programmes in your own country and why?
2. What were the strengths that PPAT brought to the implementation of HIV/AIDS prevention activities in Thailand?
3. What steps did PPAT take to try and ensure the effectiveness of their AIDS education programmes? What additional indicators might PPAT have used to evaluate this effectiveness?
4. What strategies were used by PPAT to help it maintain its effectiveness and to deal with the changes brought about by its decision to get involved in Thailand's fight against AIDS?

5. What strategies had PPAT used to finance its activities? What suggestions would you make to PPAT in relation to their future funding?

BACKGROUND

Family planning has a long history in Thailand with government services first being offered on a trial basis in 1964. By 1991, the National Family Planning Programme, supported by several NGO's, had helped to achieve a contraceptive prevalence rate of more than 60%. (Exhibit 1).

The Planned Parenthood Association of Thailand (PPAT) was founded in 1968, two years prior to official government recognition of family planning. As a private, non-proflt organisation, affiliated to the International Planned Parenthood Federation (IPPF), it operates proudly as the only family planning NGO under the patronage of Her Royal Highness the Princess Mother.

PPAT's strength lies in the Thai people. Members of the Association are drawn from all walks of life, are committed to family planning, and actively participate in PPATs activities and the annual General Assembly. From among their ranks, members elect representatives to the PPAT Council and the Executive Committee, the policy and decision-making levels of the Association. In 1992, more than 7,000 grassroots and professional volunteers were contributing to PPAT's programmes.

PPAT's mission was detined as helping to improve the quality of family life for the Thai people. (Exhibit 2) "Within this context" said the Executive Director, Khun Somphong Pattawichaiporn, "our concern is much broader than contraception alone. Although family planning remains our central focus, PPAT must be interested in anything that affects family quality, particularly among those people who are not reached by other programmes."

PPAT's Three Year Plan for 1993-1995 reflected these concerns, listing the need to improve family life and sex education for in and out-of-school adolescents to reduce the incidence of unwanted pregnancies, prostitution, STDs and divorce; to provide health and family planning information to factory workers; to provide information and services to migrant workers living in poor health and environmental conditions; and accessing those whom others find difficult to reach, such as people living in remote areas or who differ from the majority in terms of language, religion or culture.

THE START OF PPAT'S INVOLVEMENT IN AIDS PREVENTION

Reports of HIV started to reach Thailand in 1982. By 1986, despite government reluctance to allow public debate of the issue, open campaigning had started. Then the climate changed in Thailand

and a public health campaign was launched proclaiming AIDS as a deadly disease which was associated with drug use, prostitution, homosexuality and promiscuous behaviour. This created fear and discrimination against the "high-risk groups", encouraging denial among those whom the education programme most needed to help. Condoms were promoted as the key to protection against infection.

Between 1982 and 1988, PPAT followed reports on the HIV virus and AIDS. As PPAT learned about HIV and of others' attempts to fight the epidemic, it became increasingly clear that PPAT had a role to play in Thailand. PPAT also recognised the dangers inherent in the approach taken by the first public health campaign on AIDS. In 1987, an AIDS Prevention Unit was established by IPPF at its headquarters in London, and shortly afterwards PPAT sent some of its staff to attend a training programme on AIDS organised by IPPF tor the staff of its affiliates in the Asia region. By 1988, at the time of the first World AIDS day, PPAT managers and statf had discussecl and agreed on the approach that PPAT should take to the AIDS issue. Participating in the 'walkathon', the PPAT's message was that "AIDS is not so frightening if you know the facts". Following the teachings of Buddha, people should not believe what they are told to believe, but should believe because they themselves are convinced. This has formed the basis of PPAT's approach, both to family planning and to AIDS prevention.

In 1989, the Royal Thai Government called for government, NGO and other private sector agencies to collaborate in programmes for the prevention and control of HIV infection. The National Medium Term Plan for AIDS Prevention and Control then developed a framework for this collaboration, identifying the primary role of the NGOs as that of education.

EDUCATION FOR AIDS PREVENTION

(a) The General Public

Among the general population, PPAT aimed to create awareness and knowledge of population and environmental issues, family planning and health. By August 1992, PPAT's Information, Education and Motivation (IEM) programme was very busy. The eleven staff, working from a well-equipped studio, were producing 3-5 minute TV programmes for daily broadcasting by 8 national and regional TV stations.

This "Window of Life" series covered topics concerning health, FP, food and nutrition, the environment and AIDS. At the same time, IEM staff were recording 30-minute weekly radio programmes, together with shorter programmes and spots for daily broadcasting from 98 stations across the country, using local languages where appropriate. IEM staff had also produced films (such as the cartoon on the proper use of condoms), flip charts, slides, leaflets, calendars, posters, booklets, and exhibition materials on family life education, family planning, sexually-transmitted diseases (STDs) and AIDS for both the general public and for use within PPAT's projects.

IEM programme staff regularly participate in training programmes and workshops on issues related to family planning and development and IEC. In developing the AIDS education materials and programmes, the IEM staff invited HIV+ persons to visit PPAT to share their views, ideas and concerns. Wherever possible, materials are pre-tested and their effectiveness evaluated by both PPAT staff and clients. To evaluate the TV and radio programmes, staff would interview a sample of viewers and listeners. Yet another indication of effectiveness came from the number of people who followed the suggestion made during the programmes that they write to PPAT to request further information.

Although well aware of the needs in Thailand for counselling and support for those concerned about their HIV status, those identified as HIV+, and those suffering from AIDS, PPAT's policy was that IEM staff should refer those asking for help to agencies which specialised in HIV/AIDS services. All PPAT materials included details on where clients could obtain further information and professional help.

(b) Students

In collaboration with the Ministry of Education, PPAT started more than 10 years ago to promote the teaching of family life education (FLE) within secondary schools by training FLE teachers and providing teaching materials. In 1984, and with help from government health officials, information about STDs was included in the curriculum. By 1992, the project began to target students in vocational colleges and universities for FLE/AIDS education, working with both teaching staff and students. The IEM programme developed special IEM materials for use in the project and support was given to those who agreed to become peer educators among the student body. To develop the skills of the project staff in FLE and in working with youth, PPAT encouraged staff to attend relevant training programmes and seminars both within the Asia region and further a field.

(c) Out-of School Youth

Growing out of PPAT's long experience of working with slum communities on family planning, the Youth Development Services Project aimed to provide FLE/AIDS information to young people from such communities in the Bangkok area. With help from the local health centre, priority locations within the community were identified. Project staft would then approach the community leaders to explain the project and to ask for the leader's help in nominating participants to the education sessions. On the day agreed with the leader, PPAT staff and professional volunteers would meet with the selected community members to share information about AIDS, encouraging the participants to ask questions and to voice their doubts.

To support this project, PPAT developed films, posters, flipcharts and booklets which engaged people's attention and helped in communication. Pre- and post-meeting questionnaires on HIV/AIDS were completed by a sample of participants to give immediate feedback on how effectively the information had been communicated. At the end of each meeting, the participants were asked to nominate one person to become a volunteer educator for the community, to talk to others about what they had learned.

Two to three months after the meeting, PPAT would bring together several of the newly-recruited volunteers to discuss their work, to try to help them with any problems, and to provide any further information or clarification they might need. Subsequently, project members would try to keep in contact with these grassroots volunteers and to continue providing support and encouragement. The volunteers were asked to refer people who needed professional advice or treatment to a health centre.

(d) Factory Workers

In 1989, a number of NGOs were asked by the Government to carry out occupational health and family planning education for factory workers. From within the specific areas of the country that PPAT was asked to cover, project staff first identitied the larger factories (more than 50 employees) and then approached the factory owners to obtain their permission to talk to their workers. Project staff would explain the potential benefits of providing health and family planning education, including reduced absenteeism due to pregnancy, health problems and accidents. Once granted access to the workers, the project staff then had to find ways of meeting with them without affecting their earnings or production levels. The project trained worker representatives and where available, factory clinic staff, to disseminate information about family planning and STDs and to sell contraceptives. As an incentive, the volunteers kept 50% of the income from the sale of the pills and condoms supplied by PPAT.

Based on this experience, and building on their contacts and the network of factory volunteers that had already been created, in 1991 PPAT extended the scope of the project to include dissemination of information about AIDS. By August 1992, PPAT had plans to expand the project to include a larger number of factories,.

(e) Prisoners

PPAT's work with prisoners started around 1982, when it was asked by a prison social worker to give family planning information to prisoners who were about to be released.

This led to a more formal arrangement for PPAT to train medical, nursing and dental staff of the central Department of Correction, followed by the training of social workers, guards, vocational trainers and chaplains from the prisons themselves. While supporting the Department of Correction in the development of their own training team to take over responsibility for FP/AIDS education, PPAT staff also visited the prisons to talk directly to the prisoners.

The questions asked by the prisoners during these visits, led the Department of Correction to ask PPAT to include information about STDs in their talks. In 1989, information about HIV infection and AIDS was added to the programme, helped by a PPAT video developed for the prisoners, which used a comedy group to convey the AIDS messages. To reinforce the education given by officials, prison social workers would select prisoner 'volunteers', give them further training, provide them with a handbook and a chart. and encourage them to talk to their colleagues about family planning, STDs and AIDS. Support to the government on this and other projects led to a request from the Royal Thai Airforce for PPAT to provide FLE/AIDS education for their conscripts. By 1995, PPAT planned to have reached 15,000 men through video shows, discussions and printed materials.

(f) Fishermen

Thailand's fishermen play a significant role in the Thai economy. However, their working conditions and their life styles are barriers hindering their participation in national health and FP programmes. Their situation led PPAT to expand their tamily planning work to include an FLE/AIDS information component for the fishermen. Working closely with the Fishery Association, the Department of Fishery, the district health officers, and ship owners, PPAT produced a video and printed materials for the fishing communities and to disseminate the information among the fishermen and their wives through bars, special meetings and exhibitions.

(g) Clinic Services

In 1992, PPAT was providing family planning services to around 45,000 acceptors through a total of 21 clinics across the country, including some of the many refugee camps along Thailand's borders and mobile clinics to reach more remote communities. PPAT planned to open two new clinics to respond to demands for FP in cities in the East and Northeast of the country.

In all their programmes and projects, PPAT placed great emphasis on the quality of their work rather than aiming simply for greater coverage. In contrast to government facilities, clients of PPAT's clinics could make appointments and be assured of prompt service. Depending on the staff and facilities available, for a small fee the clinics provided contraceptive services (including tubectomy, vasectomy, IUD, norplant, injectables, pills and condoms), infertility treatment, pregnancy testing, ante-natal care, pap smears, STD diagnosis and treatment, and pre-marital check-ups. When requested by a client, clinic staff would provide information about HIV/AIDS, could provide counselling and, if laboratory services were available at the clinic, could provide a first HIV blood test (with client referral to a health facility for the confirmatory test). All the clinic statf had received training in HIV/AIDS. At least one nurse in each major clinic had received training in counselling either from other PPAT staff who had been sent abroad for training, or from the Thai Red Cross Society.

ORGANISATION AND MANAGEMENT

In 1992, PPAT had approved positions for 120 staff. (Exhibit 3). There was little turnover among PPAT's staff: many had been in-post for more than five years; several for more than ten. PPAT tried to maintain a stable workforce, despite its project-based funding. The salaries that PPAT could offer were a little higher than those paid for government service, but did not compete with the financial and fringe benefits offered by the private sector. The many volunteers working with PPAT consisted both of 'grassroots' volunteers from the communities and professionals from the government and private sectors who donated their time and expertise to assist in PPAT's activities.

PPAT's head office is located in Bangkok, with regional centres in Chiang Mai in the North and Khon Kaen in the Northeast. The senior managers made frequent visits to the regional offices and field-based projects to exchange information on how the work was going and to share ideas. The day-to-day operations were managed by the project leaders. A meeting of all PPAT staff and volunteers was held each year to talk about activities and plans and to reinforce the sense of partnership.

After each project activity, the responsible staft member completed a short activity report and evaluation which was reviewed by the project leader and senior managers before going to the Planning and Evaluation Unit for recording of the relevant statistics as part of PPAT's monitoring system. Beyond these more formal meetings and procedures, there was a constant exchange of information and sharing of views. As the Deputy Director, Khun Montri Pekanan said; "I hardly need to look at the activity reports, because usually I have already talked to the people involved".

In 1992, PPAT had a total of nine projects; several being implemented simultaneously in different parts of the country and some covering more than one target group. Each had a project leader and a core team of staff (Exhibit 4). Other PPAT staft would participate in the project as required and as far as their work schedule allowed. The clinic staff, tor example, might find themselves assisting the IEM programme in the design of informational materials on STDs, giving talks on family planning or leading a discussion on AIDS. The leader of the AIDS education project might one day be talking to prisoners about AIDS, another day training PPAT staff in counselling techniques, and on yet another occasion, facilitating a discussion about family planning among a group of young people in the slums. This system helped PPAT to take full advantage of individual skills and experience.

Appointment as project leader was not a permanent position. As projects ended and new ones were initiated, previous project leaders might find themselves in a supporting position on another programme where their expertise was required, while other individuals, who had demonstrated their capability and interest, might be given the opportunity to lead a new project. "Of course staff can make mistakes - we all do", said Khun Somphong, "but if something goes wrong, that's my responsibility, not their fault".

As an IPPF affiliate, PPAT received financial, material and technical support from IPPF (Exhibit 5). Only a small increase in IPPF funds had been made available to finance the HIV/AIDS activities of the FPAs. PPAT recognised that trends worldwide indicated a general decrease in donor support, particularly for those countries such as Thailand which had achieved significant economic and social advances. PPAT's Three Year Plan for 1993-1995 identified that all FPA's would have to become more self-reliant financially by increasing their income from local sources. PPAT was also wondering how it might increase the level of in-kind local contributions that it had managed to attract in the past. (Exhibit 6).

EXHIBIT 1

Demographic and Social Data On Thailand (1991)

DEMOGRAPHIC INDICATORS:	
Total Population	56.9 million
Male	28.4 million
Female	28.5 million
Married women of reproductive age (MWRA)	8.5 million
Youth (15-24)	12.2 million
Children (under 15)	18.2 million
Urban population	18.5 percent
Rural popul ation	81.5 percent
Population growth rate	1.4 percent
Crude birth rate	20.3 per 1000
Crude death rate	5.9 per 1000
Infant mortality rate	29.0 per 1000
EDUCATIONAL INDICATORS:	
Average literacy rate (age 7+)	85.1 percent
Primary school graduates entering secondary school	59.2 percent
Number of out-of-school youth	8.4 million
Number of school drop-outs	0.4 million
SOCIAL INDICATORS:	
Average age of marriage for women (1985 data)	19.7 years
Average family size	4.7 persons
Households owning radios	8.4 million
Households owning televisions	0.4 million
CONTRACEPTIVE PREVALENCE RATES:	
Total CPR (national average)	61.3 percent
Tubectomy	22.4 percent
Vasectomy	4.9 percent
Pills	16.0 percent
IUD	6.8 percent
Injectables	10.3 percent
Norplant	0.7 percent

Source: Annual Report 1991, Planned Parenthood Association of Thailand

EXHIBIT 2

OBJECTIVES (Mission Statement)

PPAT believes that knowledge of family planning is a basic human right, and that a balance between the country's population and its natural resource and productivity is a necessary condition for people's happiness, prosperity and peace.
The Association's set objectives are:

1. To promote family planning (FP) as a basic human right, along with responsible parenthood.
2. To provide extensive FP information and services to the target population groups and the general public through IE & M, clinical, training and counselling services.
3. To promote awareness of population problems and the improvement of quality of life of the Thai population.
4. To implement projects in support of the National Family Planning Policy/Programme and upon the government's special requests.
5. To cooperate, join activities and establish relationships with other governmental and private organisations both in and outside the country which share common objectives.
6. To receive and procure funds and/or contraceptives as well as other commodities and contributions in kind for use in support of the Association's family planning and other integrated development activities.

Source: PPAT Organisational Brochure.

EXHIBIT 3

Personnel Summary

Staff Assignment	Actual 1991	Approved Budget 1992	Forecast		
			1993	1994	1995
Proiects \1	81	86	90	90	94
Proiect Support	16	17	17	17	17
Administration & General	16	17	17	17	17
Total \2	113	120	124	124	128

\1 Includes: 8 doctors, 13 nurses and 13 assistant nurses for the PPAT clinics and service delivery in the refugee camps; approximately 30 programme and project staff with social science/teaching backgrounds.

\2 1991 salary costs equated to Baht 14,296,360 or 36.4% of total PPAT recurrent expenditure in 1991.

EXHIBIT - 4

Planned Parenthood Association of Thailand- Organisational Structure

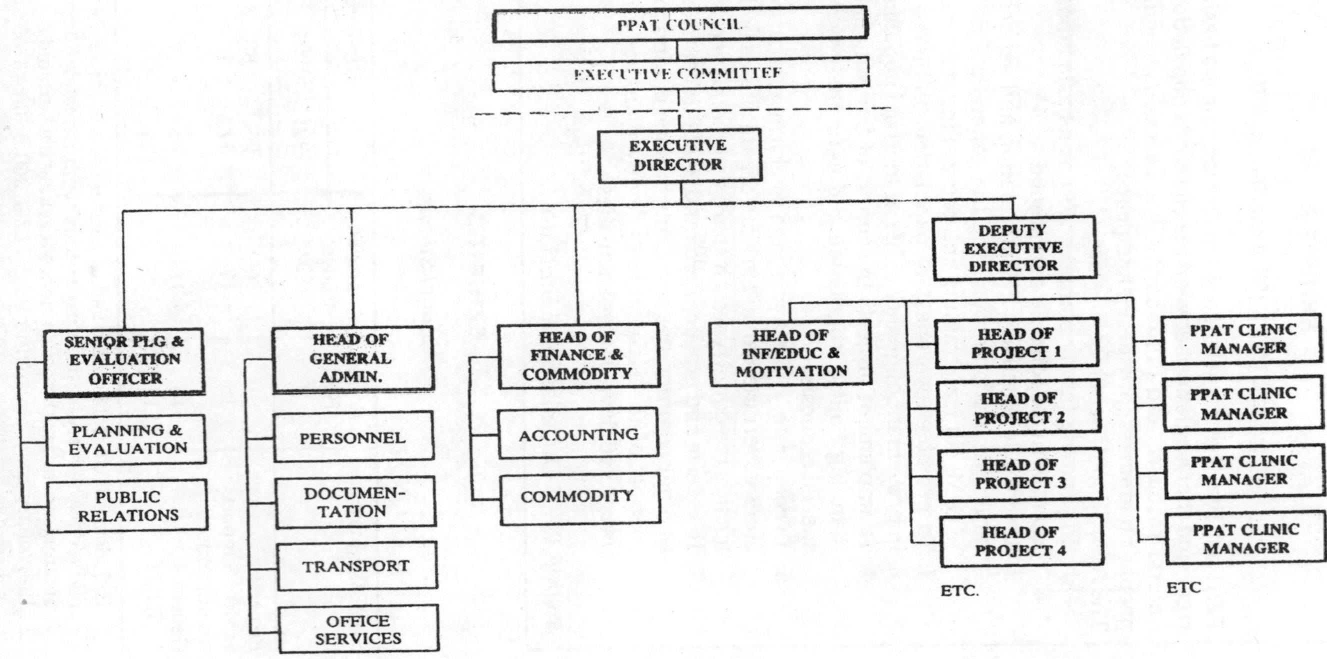

EXHIBIT -5

Income And Expenditure Summary 1991[1]

INCOME/EXPENDITURE CATEGORY		ACTUAL BUDGET 1991	APPROVED BUDGET 1992	FORECAST		
				1993	1994	1995
INCOME:	EXTERNAL SOURCES:					
	IPPF	15,274,913	15,901,900	16,556,000	17,982,000	19,696,000
	FPIA	1,677,420	1,800,000	1,800,000	1,800,000	0
	AIDAB	618,005	0	459,000	0	0
	CCT	204,201	250,000	0	0	0
	Diakonia Baptist Union/Sweden	3,505,087	3,480,000	4,880,000	1,500,000	0
	Tudor Trust & Public Welfare	772,900	0	1,200,000	0	0
	SUB-TOTAL	22,052,526	21,431,900	24,895,000	21,282,000	19,696,000
	National Sources:					
	Membership Subscriptions	10,200	10,000	10,000	10,000	10,000
	Contraccptive Sales	5,621,011	5,650,000	6,050,000	6,200,000	6,400,000
	Medical Clinic Income	7,001,420	8,700,000	8,800,000	8,900,000	9,400,000
	IEM Product Sales	54,979	70,000	70,000	80,000	80,000
	Govemment Subsidy	200,000	200,000	400,000	400,000	400,000
	FLE for Youth Project (IEM product sales)	153,007	200,000	200,000	220,000	240,000
	Govennment Funds for Hill Tribe Area Project	2,248,672	2,400,000	2,450,000	2,500,000	2,550,000
	Investment Income	2,048,896	1,200,000	1,700,000	1,700,000	1 ,700,000
	Fund Raising and Other	90,429	80,000	80,000	90,000	90,000
	SUB-TOTAL[2]	17,428,614	18,510,000	19,760,000	20,100,000	20,870,000
	TOTA INCOME [3]	39,481,140	39,941,900	44,655,000	41,382,000	40,566,000

{Cont.}...

INCOME/EXPENDITURE CATEGORY	ACTUAL BUDGET 1991	APPROVED BUDGET 1992	FORECAST		
			1993	1994	1995
EXPENDITURE: PROJECTS:					
FP Services for Low Income People	1,532,291	1,351,500	1,318,000	1,397,000	1,480,000
Comprehensive FP Services	9,090,594	8,681,000	10,265,000	10,481,000	12,409,000
Integrated Quality of Life for Rural People	1,098,458	1,154,400	1,085,000	1,150,000	1,219,000
IEM Resource Development and Campaign	2,853,401	3,001,000	2,889,000	3,062,000	3,246,000
Community-Based FLE to Southern Population	3,296,990	3,716,000	3,368,000	2,975,000	1,246,000
FP/FLE to Refugees	1 ,510,274	1 ,405,000	1,014,000	1,074,000	0
Youth Development Services	5,446,899	5,427,000	6,744,000	3,550,000	2,255,000
FP Northern Project	5,720,453	5,828,000	6,190,000	5,289,000	5,606,000
Dissemination of Knowledge on AIDS prevention	179,999	307,000	320,000	339,000	360,000
SUB-TOTAL	30,729,359	30,870,900	33,193,000	29,317,000	27,821,000
EXPENDITURE: PROJECT SUPPORT: (continued) (Includes: public relations; library services; meetings of PPAT Board; planning and evaluation; staff and volunteer development; and other administrative services directly attributable to projects.)	4,220,862	4,566,000	4,797,000	5,085,0005,	390,000

ADMINISTRATION & GENERAL SERVICES: (Includes: personnel costs; travel & per diem; materials & equipment; communications, vehicle operation and maintenance; office utilities; insurance; vehicle maintenance and operation; etc .)	4,331,540	4,500,000	4,689,000	4,970,000	5,268,000
TOTAL EXPENDITURE\3	39,261,761	39,936,900	42,679,000	39,372,000	38,479,000

\1 Figures in Thai Baht. Based on an average 1991/92 exchange rate of Baht 25.5/US$ 1. The National Bank of Thailand lists inflation rate at 5-6%.

\2 10% of locally-raised funds retained by PPAT without compromising PPAT's funding proposals to IPPF.

\3 Excludes investment income/expenditure related to procurement of contraceptives, medical supplies and equipment, and vehicles. Sources of contraceptives include imports from IPPF; IPPF-funded local purchases (where the price of local products is lower than that of the IPPF price list); and Ministry of Public Health.

Source: Planned Parenthood Association of Thailand, Three Year Plan 1993-1995.

EXHIBIT 6

IN-KIND CONTRIBUTIONS 1991-1995

INCOME/EXPENDITURE CATEGORY	ACTUAL BUDGET 1991	APPROVED BUDGET 1992	FORECAST 1993	FORECAST 1994	FORECAST 1995
SAVINGS ON RENTALS AND OTHER FEE SERVICES:					
- Free use of vehicles/drivers	434,000	500,000	431,000	427,000	428,000
- Contraceptive packaging and loading	70,000	80,000	60,000	50,000	. 50,000
- Loan of audio-visual equipment	86,000	I,100,000	92,000	92,000	93,000
- Free radio air-time	3,420,000	3,473,400	3,580,000	3,682,000	3,745,000
- Free and sponsored TV air-time	42,416,400	48,366,500	41,010,000	42,011,000	43,011,000
- Volunteered time by resource persons	50,000	50,000	50,000	50,000	50,000
- Exemptions from passport fees	10,000	12,000	12,000	12,000	12,000
- Free training rooms	43,000	1,260,000	39,000	37,000	38,000
- Trainees' per diem, registration fees & travel	416,000	365,000	406,000	337,000	338,000
DONATIONS IN-KIND:					
- Printed documents	1,137,500	995,400	I ,045,000	1,060,000	1,026,000
- Records, cassettes and video tapes	30,000	30,600	30,000	30,000	30,000
- Prizes (for fund raising)	30,000	20,000	25,000	25,000	25,000
- Food (for training/education sessions)	10,000	10,000	11,000	8,000	8,000
- Medicines, medical & chemical supplies, & vaccines	1,970,800	1,114,600	1,476,000	1,531,000	1,436,500
- Free column space for publicising PPAT	8,000,000	7,650,000	7,700,000	7,800,000	7,900,000
- Construction materials	2,000	2,000	2,000	0	0
TOTAL	58.125.700	65.029,500	55,967,000	57,152,000	58,190,500

Source: Planned Parenthood Association of Thailand, Three Year Plan 1993-1995.

FACILITATOR'S NOTES

GENERAL POINTS ABOUT USING THE CASE

1. Participants should be encouraged to read the case and to prepare their own analysis before it is discussed with others in the classroom. The discussion questions should be handed out with the case to assist participants in their analysis.
2. Generally, discussion of this case has required 1½ to 2 hours (assuming that participants have previously read the case and prepared their own analysis).
3. The discussion questions included with this case are intended to help participants to focus on what were considered to be particularly important issues illustrated in the case. However, the case may highlight many other interesting points for participants and they should be encouraged to examine, analyse and discuss these if raised.
4. The notes that follow are intended to assist the facilitator to prepare to teach the case. They provide a synopsis of the information given in the case, together with some ideas on strategies that CASP might adopt in the future. These notes should not replace the facilitator's own preparation and analysis. At all times, the facilitator should encourage the participants to reach their own conclusions, based upon a thorough analysis of the information given.
5. When introducing participants to the case, the facilitator should stress that the case is intended to facilitate discussion on important organisational and programmatic issues; it is not intended to demonstrate good or bad practices, nor to evaluate the work of PPAT. It should also be stressed that the case focuses on PPAT's HIV/AIDS activities; it does not attempt to represent the full range of PPAT's programmes.

CASE SYNOPSIS

Discussion Question 1:

What factors facilitated the addition of HIV/AIDS interventions to PPAT's family planning programmes? What additional factors might influence the integration of HIV/AIDS programmes in your own country and why?

(a) Facilitating Factors:

Despite the words of the Executive Director quoted in the case, PPAT's prime mission, as shown in Exhibit 2, is the delivery of family planning information and services. PPAT members and staff were "committed to family planning" and, in addition, this was a time when there was still widespread fear of AIDS and discrimination against those infected with the HIV virus. PPAT's clients might themselves have been "scared away" from the family planning clinics if they felt that PPAT was dealing with those infected with AIDS. Similarly, PPAT staff might have been anxious about their own reputations and the potential risks involved in working with those who might be infected. Despite these potential problems, PPAT appears to have managed the transition with few problems. Some of the possible reasons, as indicated in the Case are as follows:

- IPPF, PPAT's most important funding agent and to which PPAT was affiliated, had established its own AIDS Prevention Unit;
- By 1989, the Thai Government was changing its HIV/AIDS prevention and education strategy. At that time, it was then seeking NGO-Government collaboration in the fight against AIDS and this would have helped to justify PPAT's action with its Council and Executive Committee members;
- International reports of HIV/AIDS prevention activities and programmes would have helped PPAT to convince both its members and staff of the need for it to get involved in HIV/AIDS;
- The increasing rates of HIV infection in Thailand would also have had an impact on how PPAT members and staff viewed the problem of AIDS;
- PPAT's managers were committed to "improving the quality of life for the Thai people". Given the regular meetings and the general open communication among the staff, it is likely that this commitment would have been shared by other staff and volunteers.
- PPAT staff educated themselves through reading and discussing information and reports about HIV transmission and prevention. In addition, several staff members attended training events and conferences on HIV/AIDS (such as the IPPF HIV/AIDS training programme for FPA staff. This would have helped staff to understand how HIV was transmitted and to reduce their own fears.
- PPAT encouraged staff members to discuss the situation and contribute to the decision about the course of action PPAT should take.
- PPAT made a gradual movement towards a decision (from 1982 to 1988).

(b) Factors that might influence HIV/AIDS and FP integration in other countries:

- Family planning might not be as well accepted as it clearly was in Thailand. Adding HIV/AIDS interventions to the family planning activities might be seen as threatening the effectiveness of the family planning efforts.
- Whilst family planning may be acceptable in some countries for married couples, the provision of sex education, counselling, and talking openly about STDs and safer-sex practices, might be very difficult. Public (and therefore, official) sentiment would therefore be opposed to any HIV/AIDS education and services being offered outside of the faniily planning clinic.
- Religious barriers might hinder the promotion of condoms for STD protection among unmarried couples, since this would be viewed as 'promoting promiscuous behaviour'.
- HIV infection levels might be perceived as less of a threat than in Thailand, so both family planning clients and staff might not accept the need to provide HIV prevention education or services.
- A government's position on HIV/AIDS (whether it recognises AIDS as a problem; whether it is willing to talk openly about the risks to everyone and how people can protect themselves; whether it has established any programmes either within the government agencies or through nongovernmental organisations) will also have a significant influence on how a family planning programme will respond.
- Donors often differentiate between condoms provided tor family planning and those supplied to a country for HIV/AIDS services. A family planning programme might find itself in difficulties with its donors over the reasons for its promotion of condom use.
- The extent to which the family planning programme already offers other related services such as screening for cervical cancer, gynaecological examinations and treatment, STD services, etc. will probably have a significant influence on the ease with which HIV/AIDS interventions can be added to the portfolio of activities.

Discussion Question 2:

What were the strengths that PPAT brought to the implementation of HIV/AIDS prevention activities in Thailand ?

- PPAT was a well-established and well-respected Thai organisation, as evidenced by its 24-year history, the patronage of Her Royal Highness, the collaboration with Government agencies and the size of its volunteer network.
- PPAT had more than 7000 grass-roots and professional volunteers already active in promoting family planning information and services.
- PPAT already had extensive contacts with those communities which, for reasons of lifestyle, income levels, living and working conditions, might suffer disproportionately from HIV infection and yet might be the hardest for government services to reach and influence.
- As an integral part of its tamily planning education, counselling and services, PPAT staff already had experience of talking to clients about sexuality and sexual behaviour.
- Family planning clients represent those who are most in need of information about HIV protection.
- PPAT's clinic services already included diagnosis and treatment of STDs, together with pre-marital counselling and check-ups. This gave them the opportunity to build HIV/AIDS information into their services.

Discussion Question 3:

What steps did PPATtake to try and ensure the effectiveness of theirAIDS education programmes? What additional indicators might PPAT have used to evaluate this effectiveness?

(a) Steps taken by PPAT:

- PPAT kept in contact with the experiences of HIV/AIDS programmes in other countries, learning about effective (and ineffective approaches) to prevention.
- The meetings with HIV+ individuals to develop PPAT's own understanding of the issues involved and the concerns and needs of those infected.
- The extensive use of radio programmes and spots, together with the more restricted use of television programmes to disseminate HIV/AIDS information clearly matched the data on the availability of the radios and TVs in Thailand. (Exhibit 1) Similarly, high literacy rates enabled PPAT to make extensive use of written materials in its education programmes.

- The pre-testing of IEM materials and programmes.
- Interviews with viewers and listeners following airing of the TV and radio programmes.
- The letters from listeners/viewers asking for further information after the programmes.
- Development of targetted IEM materials for the different groups with whom PPAT was working (i.e. students, out-of-school youth, prisoners, fishermen and factory workers).
- The pre and post-meeting questionnaires administered to the participants at the HIV/AIDS education sessions among the slum communities.
- The follow-up of the peer-educators drawn from the slum communities and the provision of continued support and reinforcement for their work.

(b) Other Possible Indicators of Effectiveness:

- Requests from teaching staff at the schools and colleges to provide further information.
- Reports from the various peer educators about the frequency and the types of questions they are asked relating to HIV/AIDS.
- The numbers of condoms sold by the factory representatives prior to and following the inclusion of HIV/AIDS int'ormation in the workers' education programme.
- The conduct of KAP stuclies among the communities with which PPAT was working might have provided further indications of the impact of their education programmes.

Discussion Question 4:

What strategies were used by PPAT to help it maintaine its effectiveness and to deal with the changes brought about by its decision to get involved in Thailand 's fight against AIDS?

- PPAT's style of management, as inclicated in the case, was both open and supportive. This would have encouraged staff and volunteers to voice and discuss their concerns and doubts and to work these through with their colleagues.
- The stability of PPAT's workforce indicated a general satisfaction with the organisation and its work. One could also assume that this stability indicates mutual trust between the managers and staff which would facilitate organisational change and development.

- Communication was clearly important to PPAT: the senior PPAT managers made frequent visits to the field to keep in contact both with the individuals and the programmes; informal discussions and sharing of information took place all the time. This would have helped to keep the managers in touch with the staff views and contributed to building a sense of teamwork.
- PPAT's approach to the allocation of work to staff members would have helped to ensure that many individuals would have the opportunity to work on the HIV/AIDS education programmes and thereby experience first hand both the communities' needs for information and their response to PPAT's programmes. This would help to develop understanding among the staff. The system would also have helped to maintain individual's interest in their jobs and to develop their skills.
- PPAT's HIV/AIDS interventions all grew out of their existing or previous programmes and PPAT built upon its contacts and its relationships with the communities. This should have made the clients more receptive to PPAT's HIV/AIDS education activities and helped PPAT in deciding on approaches that would be both acceptable and effectively.
- PPAT had clearly managed to maintain a clear focus and mission. The annual meetings between the staff and volunteers, the fact that many staff have stayed with PPAT despite the availability of higher salaries within the private sector, and the fact that it had managed to integrate HIV/AIDS education activities into so many of its programmes and projects, were all evidence that PPAT had managed a significant programme change successfully and effectively.

Discussion Question 5:

What strategies had PPAT used to finance its activities? What suggestions would you make to PPAT in relation to their future funding?

(a) Strategies used for financing:

- In addition to IPPF, PPAT was receiving funds from five other external sources. This would have involved making contact with the funding organisations to establish their interest and the development of project proposals and budgets. It is also significant that each of these external donors had committed funds for at least two years (Exhibit 5 does not tell us when these projects funds were first made available).

- PPAT also received Government funding for the Hill Tribe Area Project, thus indicating that it is providing services to a community that the Government finds difficult to reach effectively.

- Other local sources of cash included sales of contraceptives and IEM materials, income derived from clinic service charges, membership fees and special fund raising events. Significant interest income was also derived from investment of funds.

- Contributions and donations in-kind are impressive (Exhibit 6), although participants might question how PPAT costed these. It also appears that PPAT might have negotiated some long-term agreements with the various contributors, or at least had sufficient confidence that the contributions would continue to be forthcoming over the following three years.

(b) Suggestions regarding future funding:

- All of the external sources of income (excluding IPPF) will be completed by 1995. Given the usual lead time for donors to commit new funds, PPAT needs to start an early search for new sources of programme support. The case indicates that external funding sources for Thailand, may be difficult to locate and this adds to the urgency. PPAT might be advised to search for donors interested in supporting HIV/AIDS projects as opposed to the traditional FP donors. Whatever the strategy chosen by PPAT to identify new external sources of funding, PPAT needs to 'parcel' its planned future activities, such that proposals can be developed for individual potential donors.

- PPAT might review its schedule of fees for clinic services, contraceptives, IEM materials and membership dues to establish whether these could reasonably be raised without affecting the volume of sales or client demands. Alternatively, PPAT might establish different schedules of fees for clinic services, depending on the location of the clinic and its clientele.

- Additional eft'orts on special fund-raising events might be considered, since income from this source appears minimal.

- PPAT might also consider the potential for charging small fees for the factory worker education progrargmes or starting new worker education programmes in larger companies in the Bangkok at other major urban areas.

4

Commercial Blood Donors and AIDS Prevention

THE GUJARAT AIDS PREVENTION UNIT, AHMEDABAD

RADIUM BHATTACHARYA
JENNY HUDDART
DONNA BJERRGAARD
GLEN WILLIAM

NOTES ON USING THE CASE

1. In addition to these notes, the materials relating to the Planned Parenthood Association of Thailand consist of:
   (a) Learning Objectives;
   (b) Discussion Questions;
   (c) The Case;
   (d) Facilitators' Notess
2. The discussion questions are intended to help readers to focus on what are considered to be particularly important issues illustrated in the Case. However, the Case may highlight other interesting points and you are encouraged to examine, analyse and discuss these with others.
3. You should review the Objectives and Discussion Questions before turning to the Case itself. After reading the Case carefully, you should then return to the Discussion Questions and prepare your own responses to these, making notes as appropriate, before discussing the case with others.

4. Doing something oneself is the most effective method of learning. Therefore, to get the maximum bepefit from the Case, you should prepare your own analysis of the Case before comparing this with points raised in the Facilitators' Notes.
5. There are no right or wrong answers to the Discussion Questions posed. The important issue is the ability to analyse the factors that are influencing the situation and the use of this analysis to draw conclusions about the future.
6. The case is intended to facilitate discussion on important organisational and programmatic issues; it is not intended to demonstrate good or bad practices, nor to evaluate the work of the organisation represented.

Objectives

1. To identify the environmental and organisational factors that can influence the successful design and implementation of HIV/AIDS interventions.

2. To examine the ways in which an NGO can gain the trust and cooperation of client communities in the implementation of HIV/AIDS programmes and projects.

3. To identify and evaluate the strategies that NGOs can use to promote the sustainability of their programs and projects.

Discussion Questions

1. What were the most important factors that led to the implementation of the Gujarat AIDS Prevention Unit?

   It might be helpful to consider this question in terms of:

   (a) factors relating to SIRMCE as an organisation;
   (b) factors relating to the problems the project was planning to address;
   (c) factors relating to potential support for the project.

2. What were the important things that the project did to gain the trust and confidence of those involved in the city's blood collection industry? What impact did this have on the success of the project?
3. What strategies might have helped the GAP Unit to avoid the situation that they are now in with regard to funding and the continuation of the project activities?

4. What do you see as the major strengths that the GAP Unit can offer in relation to HIV/AIDS projects and programmes in India? What suggestions could you make to Dr. Bhattacharya as she considers the GAP's future activities?

HOW IT ALL BEGAN

In 1992, I was the President of SIRMCE, India which was based in Ahmedabad. SIRMCE is the International Society for Research on Civilisation Diseases and on Environment which had its headquarters in Luxembourg. At that time we had around 100 members, including doctors, scientists, architects, engineers and planners, representing a wide range of government, non-govermnental and private sector organisations. Working with many local organisations - such as the Consumers' Education and Research Centre, Womens' groups, the Rotary and Lions Clubs, and the National Design Institute, we focussed mainly on research and advocacy related to environmental health issues such as hypertension, diabetes, obesity, and the effects of pollutants. Until the Gujarat AIDS Prevention Unit was started, we had no salaried staff, but relied on our members to volunteer their time whenever the need arose.

In 1988, members of SIRMCE were started by a report in a local newspaper which said that some HIV infected blood products were on the local market and that a few individuals had been infected by these products. We met with the Drug Controller of Gujarat State and the Consumers' Education and Research Centre, and then sent a report of the meeting to the State Government.

Soon we began to get other reports about HIV in Gujarat State and one in particular caught our attention; it stated that of 475 commercial blood donors who were screened, 420 were found to be HIV+. Although we later found that the figures were exaggerated, the situation was very worrying. A group of SIRMCE members began to meet regularly to monitor reports and discuss the situation.

In 1989, I was in London attending an international seminar and mentioned our concerns in Gujarat to a person at the seminar who offered to help us fund support. She put me in contact with IPPF/London and this led to an agreement that IPPF would fund and provide consultancy services for a 2-day workshop in Gujarat on AIDS Awareness and Prevention. This workshop, held in mid-1990, was attended by specialists from all over India who were involved in HIV surveillance or prevention programmes. During the workshop, participants developed a plan of action, together with a number of project proposals. One of these was our proposal for AIDS awareness activities among commercial blood donors in Ahmedabad.

THE COMMERCLAL BLOOD DONOR SYSTEM

In 1990, the buying and selling of blood in India was a highly developed industry. Private pathology laboratories collected and paid for blood from the individual donors and sold it to the hospitals and clinics. Despite the risks involved in the commercial blood donation system, India could not afford to stop this practice since about halt the blood used in large urban hospitals was collected in this way. In the State of Gujarat, commercial blood donors accounted for 30% of the total blood supply, and the State Government estimated that 28% of this blood was HIV-positive. The blood collection system in Ahmedabad was somewhat different from other Indian cities since the commercial blood donors could sell their blood without going through any HIV screening tests. In 1990, there were only two centres in Ahmedabad which were screening blood for HIV.

Commercial blood donors were a group particularly at risk of being infected with HIV. The virus could be transmitted through the use of the unsterilized equipment in blood collection centres, and also by unprotected sex. Contaminated blood could then quickly spread the virus to the blood recipient, to sex partners of the infected person, to other donors (through the use of unsterilised needles), to blood products, and to the foetuses of pregnant women who received transfusions.

THE PROJECT

Due to the threat that the commercial blood donation system posed to the population of Ahmedabad, SIRMCE proposed to start a scheme to help protect the blood used in the city from infection with HIV. To help develop the proposal, SIRMCE invited a number of blood donor agents (people who act as middlemen between the individual donors and the blood collection centres) to join them for the proposal development phase of the workshop. We believed that these agents could help us to understand the situation of the blood donors and to give us access to the individuals with whom we needed to work. We also realised that if the project was to be effective, we needed to have the cooperation of these agents. The agents were very helpful. For example, it was they who suggested that the project also needed to protect the blood donors themselves from infection. At the workshop, we developed the goals and outlined the activities for the project. (See Exhibit 1)

The British Overseas Development Administration agreed to finance the project, through IPPF, for a period of 18 months and we received the first funds in June 1990. To implement the plan, we established the Gujarat AIDS Prevention Unit (GAP) in December 1990, with a paid staff of five persons (a project manager, two social workers, a microbiologist and a secretary), supported by six volunteers. We also set up a small laboratory which could carry out sero-surveillance and pre- and post-test counselling.

WORKING WITH THE BLOOD DONORS

Before developing an educational programme for people who sold their blood for a living, we felt that it was essential to understand their environment, lifestyle and working conditions. With the help of the agents, we carried out a three-month study in Ahmedabad, based on interviews with 100 commercial blood donors. The study revealed that commercial blood donors were unaware of the existence of HIV and AIDS, and knew nothing about how HIV is transmitted. They were equally ignorant about sexually transmitted diseases (STDs) or how to practice safe sex. We also learned that these people often started selling their blood almost by accident. V/hen a young, illiterate man comes to the city in search of a job, he might meet someone on the street who tells him how he can earn money by selling his blood.[1]

Once they began donating their blood, commercial donors realised it was an easy way to earn a living, and became addicted to that way of lite. Some gave blood as often as ten times a month. This made them physically weak, immobile and indolent. They ate in small restaurants near their "home" on the pavement, where a meal cost only about five Rupees (US$0.20). At other times they got food from religious organisations. Slowly they lost their desire to work.

After our initial fact-gathering study, we set up the blood screening centre to provide voluntary testing of donors for HIV antibodies. We also gave pre-test counselling to inform the donors about HIV/AIDS and the chances of being infected through unsterile equipment at blood collection centres and through their own risk habits. We then issued identity cards (with photographs) to those who were HIV-free at the time of screening. Testing was repeated at three-month intervals to further ensure the safety of the donor blood. We also made contact with the collection centres to tell them about the new system that we had developed and encouraged them to accept blood only from card-holding donors.

By March 1992, the number of commercial blood donors being regularly screened had grown from the initial 100 to 433 persons, of whom 20 had tested positive for HIV - a prevalence rate of 6% . The blood donors who tested HIV negative were aware that their good health was essential to their continued ability to sell their blood and preserve their livelihood. We also found that the identity card helped the blood donors (who tended to have lost their sense of self in the big city) to confirm their existence and it gave them a new hope in their lives. They carried their card with pride.

/1 *For example, Bharat is a young mum who started selling his blood about 12 months ago. He lost his parents when he was ten years old and his eWer brother could tlOt take proper care of him. Bharat dropped out of school and did odd jobs in the village. Then he quarrelled with his brother and left the village, moving from place to place until he settled in w4hmedabad. At the age of 20 he had no money, no home, no job, and nothing to eat. One day he met Vijay, who told him he could make money by selling his blood. He has done so regularly ever since.*

Those who tested positive became part of our post-test counselling programme, and they all agreed that they would no longer sell or donate blood. They understood their responsibility to the community, and that their blood would help to spread HIV and AIDS even further.[2] We also encouraged them to become peer educators and we held weekly meetings at our office to discuss topics such as HIV and STDs and how they are transmitted; the rights of commercial blood donors; the hazards of repeated donations; condom usage; and the importance of proper nutrition, health and hygiene.

Growing out of our experience, we then had plans to try to help those commercial blood donors who had tested HIV positive and who needed to find other means of earning money. One idea was to provide vocational training to help them to develop new income generating skills. Anotber plan was to help the blood donors to establish a cooperative blood banking system through which blood could be collected from people irrespective of their HIV status. The blood could then be screened and seropositive samples sold to research organisations involved in developing vaccines: The HIV-free blood would be sold to pharmaceutical laboratories.

WORKING WITH THE BLOOD COLLECTION CENTRES

After setting up the voluntary screening and education programme for blood donors, we then concentrated our efforts on the blood collection centres themselves. We surveyed 75 registered pathology laboratories in Ahmedabad, most of which served as blood collection centres in direct contact with the city's private hospitals and health clinics. The survey revealed that HIV awareness among laboratory personnel[3] was nil and most of the laboratories did not follow the official infection control guidelines or instructions for handling body fluids.

We then began running training courses for technicians and unskilled staff, and by March 1992 had trained 30 of each. We planned

/2 *Manirum Singh, for example, came from Delhi. He was a mason by trade with a secondary school education. He knew about HIV/AIDS and said that in the State of Uttar Pradesh there were blood banks where HIV-positive donors' photograps were pasted on the walls. These donors simply move on to another city to sell their blood. Manirum Singh came to our clinic asking for the identity card which we issued to donors whose blood tested HIVnegative. Unfortunately, Maniram 's blood tested seropositive. He accepted the fact quietly, without any show of emotion. He agreed to join us as a peer educator, and even volunteered to set up a union of blood donors to ensure they were not exploited by the commercial blood banks. He said: "Who knows, I might have contracted the infection from the blood donation centre itself not During the post-test counselling session he said that since he knew his blood was infected, he did not want to sell his blood anymore. But if he stopped selling his blood he would have to look for some other way of earning money. This was a problem for other HIV+ commercial blood donors.*

/3 *Centres are usually staffed by one pathologist, two technicians and three unskilled personnel, who collect blood at a rate of one to ten units per day.*

to run a special course for pathologists at a later date. The training was designed to inform participants about HIV/AIDS and to emphasise the precautions they should take to prevent accidental infection - either of themselves or of their clients. Slide shows and wall charts were used to encourage discussion. Eventually, we planned to recruit peer educators from this group.

OTHER RELATED ACTIVITIES

As well as working to improve the safety of the blood supply in Ahmedabad, the GAP Unit saw the need to improve the conditions of the city's blood banks. We were also making a proposal to UMCEF to work with sex workers, their children and clients in Surat to educate them about health, nutrition, STDs/AIDS and safer sex practices. GAP staff had approached trade unions and the Gujarat Chambers of Commerce to brief them and their members on STDs and HIV/AIDS, and had begun working with the staff of the STD clinics of Employees' State Insurance Scheme Hospitals in the city to provide HIV/AIDS information and training.

Earlier in 1992, I had attended a meeting in Bangalore where a number of NGOs working in the field of HIV/AIDS had agreed on the need to form a national NGO network to share information and experience. We needed to make sure that we were all giving the same messages regarding HIV/AIDS, and we needed to offer each other help and support. I had realised that such a network needed to be replicated at the State level, so I was intending to find ways of linking up the 200 or so NGOs in Gujarat and to organise a meeting later in the year.

THE FUTURE

We were at the beginning of a very long journey towards AIDS prevention and control in India, but the achievements of the Gujarat AIDS Prevention Unit had been encouraging and significant, even if modest, in the national context. The programme had helped to ensure a safe blood supply as well as protecting commercial blood donors from HIV infection at blood collection centres. We were aware that it was not possible for a small NGO to take permanent responsibility for the voluntary blood screening of the donors, but we hoped that the Government might take the cue from this beginning and might replicate our project on a much larger scale.

But the funding from TPPF was coming to an end on March 21, 1992 and many of our activities could not be continued without salaried staff. As the end of the project drew closer, we approached other donors, but did not yet know if they could help - or when. "I felt so bad about this and so responsible for what has happened", said Dr. Bhattacharya.

EXHIBIT 1

The Gujarat AIDS Prevention Unit (Gap)

Project Goals

1. To help ensure a safe blood supply to the people of Ahmedabad.
2. To protect commercial blood donors from HIV infection through unsterile equipment and procedures at the blood collection centres, and through other risk behaviours such as unprotected sexual intercourse.
3. To protect the personnel working in blood collection centres from accidental infection with HIV in the course of their work.

Protject Activities

The plan that SIRMCE developed for the GAP consisted of 5 sets of activities:

1. The education of commercial blood donors about safe blood donating and how to practice safer sex.
2. The voluntary testing of commercial blood donors for HIV infection, accompanied by pre and post-test counselling.
3. Helping commercial blood donors to find alternative income generating opportunities.
4. Upgrading the existing infection prevention guidelines in commercial blood collecting centres.
5. Educating the staff at blood collection centres about the possibility of accidental transmission.

FACILITATORS' NOTES

GENERAL POINTS ABOUT USING THE CASE

1. Participants should be encouraged to read the case and to prepare their own analysis before it is discussed with others in the classroom. The discussion questions should be handed out with the case to assist participants in their analysis.

2. Generally, discussion of this case has required 1½ to 2 hours (assuming that participants have previously read the case and prepared their own analysis).

3. The discussion questions included with this case are intended to help participants to focus on what were considered to be particularly important issues illustrated in the case. However, the case may highlight many other interesting points for participants and they should be encouraged to examine, analyse and discuss these, if raised.

4. The notes that follow are intended to assist the facilitator to prepare to teach the case. They provide a synopsis of the information given in the case, together with some ideas on strategies that SIAAP might adopt in the future. These notes should not replace the facilitator's own preparation and analysis. At all times, the facilitator should encourage the participants to reach their own conclusions, based upon a thorough analysis of the information given.
5. When introducing participants to the case, the facilitator should stress that the case is intended to facilitate discussion on important organisational and programmatic issues; it is not intended to demonstrate good or bad practices, nor to evaluate the work of SIRMCE.

CASE SYNOPSIS

Discussion Question 1:

What do you think were the most important factors that led to the implementation of the Gujarat AIDS Prevention Unit? It might be helpful to consider this question by thinking of: (a) factors relating to SIRMCE as an organisation; (b) factors relating to the problems the project was planning to address; and (c) factors relating to potential support for the project.

(a) Factors relating to SIRMCE as an organisation:

- SIRMCE's members had been interested in HIV/AIDS for a couple of years before the project started.
- SIRMCE's members were clearly a committed group with a strong social conscience, as shown by their action following the newspaper reports of HIV-infected vaccines. As they learned more ahout HIV infection and AIDS through their discussions, they would also have begun to understand the risks for the comtnunity - and they themselves - faced if the local blood supply were contaminated.
- SIRMCE already had links into the community from their previous programmes. For example, with womens' organisations, consumer groups, and the Rotary and Lions Clubs.
- SIRMCE had international connections (through SIRMCE/ Luxembourg and through attending international seminars), so the members would have a good idea of the potential impact of HIV/AIDS on India and the potential rates of spread through the blood donor system.

(b) Factors relating to the problems the project was planning to address:

- A contaminated blood supply would be seen as a serious problem by the community, by the clinicians themselves and by those in positions of authority, since it could affect any one of them or their families.
- There has been a lot of attention given worldwide to protection of blood supply; this is seen as a priority by governments and donors and the actions that can be taken are relatively simple as compared to trying to change the sexual behaviours of individuals.
- The only potential 'losers' in this programme were the blood donors themselves. Everyone else (i.e. blood collection laboratories, the hospitals and the potential blood transfusion recipients) would gain from an uncontaminated blood supply. Therefore, the project would be likely to get cooperation from most parties, but had to deal carefully with the commercial blood donors to get their support.
- It might be useful for participants to identify the different groups who might be affected by the GAP programme, to assess whether the impact would be negative or positive and, against this analysis, to examine the strategies that GAP used.

(c) Factors relating to potential support for the project:

- Local donors, such as the Rotarians and Lions Club members of SIRMCE, had already shown their interest in the problem of an HIV-infected blood supply back in 1988, and SIRMCE had then established a special group to monitor the situation.
- IPPF had already shown their interest in supporting SIRMCE's activities in HIV/AIDS by agreeing to provide funds and a consultant to support the AIDS awareness and prevention workshop. SIRMCE's proposal for the project was developed at that workshop, so IPPF would have had an even greater incentive to help in its implementation.

Discussion Question 2:

What were the important steps that the project designers took to gain the trust and confidence of those involved in the city 's blood collection industry? What impact did this have on the success of the project?

- The GAP Unit involved the blood donor agents (the middlemen) right from the start by inviting them to the workshop and asking them to help design the project. This ensured that the agents were aware of the needs and the objectives of the project, that their experience and knowledge influenced the design of the project, and that they would have a sense of ownership of the project. It also gave the GAP Unit easy access to the commercial blood donors themselves.

- The study done to investigate the situation of the blood donors before the detailed project activities were decided upon was very important. By talking to the commercial blood donors the project staff gained an understanding of how the blood system worked, and of the needs and motivations of the blood donors themselves. On their side, the blood donors would have begun to get to know the project staff, and could have shared their own views of what might be done and what would be important to them.
- The system of identity cards for HIV-free donors seems to have worked in this case. It provides a motivation for the donors to be regularly tested (so that they can maintain their livlihood). But there are clearly potential dangers which could be explored with participants, for example:
  - (a) HIV-positive donors might find it difficult to maintain their anonymity in a small community where presumably the blood donors know each other and the agents well;
  - (b) There is nothing to stop the HIV+ donors from moving to another city (although GAP claims this has never yet happened);
  - (c) there is some potential for forgery (although GAP has recently started a system of changing the colour of the cards every few months and at the same time ensuring that a range of signatures are required on the cards).
- The GAP staff also carried out a survey of the blood collection laboratories - again this gave the staff of these laboratories a chance to learn about the project and its aims, and to contribute their views on what could be done to improve the situation. The training of staff would have been welcomed since it was designed in part to help them protect themselves. The donor identity card system would also have been attractive to them since it offered them a no-cost way of protecting their reputation.

Discussion Question 3:

What strategies might have helped the GAP Unit to avoid the situation that they were in with regard to funding and the continuation of the project activities?

- Since the GAP Unit was aware from the start that IPPF funding was "seed money" only and would only cover 18 months, the officers might have:
  - (a) Included, as one of their project goals, the need to find ways to cover project costs in the future. This would have kept this issue on their day-to-day agenda;
  - (b) Appointed a SIRMCE/GAP member to take responsibility for seeking project funding and other forms of support.
  - (c) Explored the potential of the private pathology laboratories carrying the cost of the training of their staff or even of establishing their own blood screening facilities;
  - (d) Explored with the authorities of the city of Ahmedabad (or used the press or other means of bringing pressure to bear) the need to change the legislation regarding blood screening, to bring the city more in line with other parts of the country and to force all blood collection laboratories to screen or get proof of screening.
  - (e) Tried to encourage the Government to take over responsibility for blood screening.
  - (f) Explored linkages with other NGO or Government programmes in Ahmedabad and the State of Gujarat to help in such areas as vocational training for HIV+ blood donors.
  - (g) Made early contact with other local or international donors to seek further support.
  - (h) Prepared short reports on the project - its activities, progress and future ideas - and shared this report with other agencies.

Discussion Question 4:

What do you see as the major strengths that the GAP Unit could offer in relation to HIV/AIDS projects and programmes in India? What suggestiolls could you make to Dr. Bhattacharya as she considers the GAP's future activities?

(a) Major strengths:

- SIRMCE's diverse and influential membership.
- Its previous experience in health areas affecting people's day to day working lives.
- Its contacts and experience with local employers and government agencies.
- The GAP Unit's growing links with local and international organisations working in HIV/AIDS .

(b) Suggested Future Strategies:

- Keep issues of sustainability on the agenda from the very start. If possible, give an individual specific responsibility for this.
- With a mainly voluntary workforce, SIRMCE needs to focus its efforts carefully. Too many activities or too diverse a programme will probably mean that little gets done, that what gets done is short-lived or superficial, and that members get less satisfaction from their work. (Refer to the GAP Unit's plans for future activities.)
- Network with other NGOs. Look for opportunities to collaborate with them, such as joint or linked programmes.
- GAP should not take on activities that some other organisation is already involved in, or is better placed to do, unless there is very good reason.
- Talk to potential donors regularly, see what their interests are and keep them informed about GAP's own plans and activities.
- Keep in contact with the local business sector and always look for opportunities to collaborate with them on activities. This will help on sustainability issues as well as provide other benefits.

5

Klong Toey: Facing Up to AIDS in a Bangkok Slum

The Work of the Duang Prateep Foundation

PART—I

Discussion Questions

1. What strategies did Duang Prateep use to try and match its HIV/AIDS activities to the needs of the community?
2. How did Duang Prateep assess the etfectiveness of its AIDS programme and how were the results of the assessments used to improve its programmes? What suggestions could you make on other ways in which Duang Prateep might evaluate its programmes?
3. What recommendations would you make to Duang Prateep on the activities and the approaches it might use in the future as it expands its AIDS programme to a further nine Klong Toey communities?

DUANG PRATEEP'S AIDS PROGRAMME

The Duang Prateep Foundation was established in 1979 by Prateep Ungsongtham, who was born in Klong Toey and worked on the docks trom the age of 12 to put herself through secondary school at night. In April 1992, the Foundation had over 100 staff members, most of whom had been recruited from the Klong Toey community itself. There was also a large network of Klong Toey volunteers who helped Duang Prateep to run its wide range of educational and community development programmes, including kindergartens, educational sponsorship, vocational training, income generation, an anti-drugs campaign and the latest addition, an AIDS prevention programme. The variety of their programmes helped Duang Prateep staff and volunteers in their HIV/AIDS work since they could visit members of the communities without fear of breaching confidentiality or causing undue embarassment. The community was involved in the administration of most of the programmes.

It was through their Freedom From Drug Abuse programme, which began in 1986, that Duang Prateep first became aware of the rapid spread of HIV in Klong Toey. In May 1988, the programme tested a group of IDUs who had been sent by the community for inpatient drug treatment and were shocked to find that 75% tested HIV-positive. Realising the potential impact of AIDS on the community, and in view of the low priority given to AIDS by the government at that time, Duang Prateep decided to start a two-year pilot programme in three of the Klong Toey communities.

Duang Prateep started by educating themselves and key members of the community about HIV/AIDS. With the assistance of Family Health International (U.S. based organisation), a seminar was held for members of the Foundation, community leaders and the police. At the seminar it was agreed that the overall aim of the AIDS programme should be prevention of HIV infection. Three target groups were identified as priorities for interventions: all members of the three communities; all IDUs, especially those known to be HIV+ and their families; and sex workers. The specific objectives were defined as: (a) to teach people how to protect themselves and their families from infection; (b) to promote understanding rather than fear of people who are HIV+; (c) to enable seropositives to live in a supportive community.

Following this seminar, the AIDS programme staff were given further training in the transmission and prevention of HIV infection and in counselling. But Duang Prateep recognised that the best education that people can have is by learning from their own experiences. So the AIDS programme staff met regularly as a group - first monthly, then weekly - to discuss their experiences, what they had learned from them, and how to use this learning to make their activities more effective. The four main programme activities during the pilot phase were as follows:

INJECTING DRUG USERS:

When the first group of 169 IDUs agreed to be tested for HIV, information was also collected on their residence, family situation, age and sex. It was found that 4 out of 5 of the youngest age group (less than 20 years) were HIV+ . There were also significant differences in the prevalence rates between the three communities. Further investigation revealed that the higher rates in one community might be explained by two factors. IDUs in this area tended to live together, so increasing the likelihood of needle-sharing. Secondly, most of the dealers lived in this neighbourhood, and as the IDUs tended to use dealer-supplied needles and as these needles were often used by other drug users, this also increased the chances of spreading Infectlon.

Armed with this information, the programme tried to recruit former IDUs as peer educators, but failed because the ex-IDUs were reluctant to let others know that they had once used drugs. The programme then decided to use Duang Prateep staff to make regular home visits to the IDUs, to give information about HIV infection and AIDS, to teach them methods of prevention including the cleaning of syringes and needles, and the use of condoms. They also provided supplies of condoms and bleach. The home visits were reinforced by encouraging small groups of IDUs (and sometimes their families) to meet at Duang Prateep to talk about their experiences and their concerns, and to provide them with opportunities to ask questions. Both the nonjudgemental attitudes of the staff and these meetings helped enormously to build up trust between the addicts and the programme.

Duang Prateep was convinced that if they were to encourage people to stop using drugs and to reduce behaviours that can lead to AIDS, they must help the IDUs to develop some hope for the future. "Filling them with a lot of 'don't do this' instructions" was unlikely to motivate them to make the necessary changes in their life unless they were also provided with alternative strategies for survival. To do this, the programme also provided vocational training for the IDUs and made small, interest-free loans available to them to develop income generating activities.

In 1990, a little over a year atter the programme started, a second survey was carried out among the IDUs in the pilot communities to collect data that would help improve the programme. The survey looked at the age at which the IDUs began using drugs (the highest proportion was found to be between 15-19 years), the amount of money spent on drugs as compared to the earnings of the IDUs (drug costs were found to exceed income), the extent to which the IDUs used drugs in groups, and the sexual habits of the IDUs (none used condoms, although several visited prostitutes). These findings led to a stronger emphasis on educating the IDUs about cleaning their equipment, more efforts to promote the use of condoms, and an understanding that attention needed to be given to the design of drug and HIVprevention strategies for children and adolescents. The data also increased the fears that IDUs, both male and female, were increasingly turning to commercial sex work to earn the money for heroin. The need to continue to help IDUs to find jobs was reinforced.

THE COMMERCIAL SEX WORKERS

In 1990, the programme used the police to encourage local brothel owners to send their sex workers to a training seminar to learn about HIV/AIDS and how to protect themselves. It also explored strategies that could be used to get the clients to use condoms. All the sex workers were tested for HIV and completed a questionnaire about AIDS.

Twenty percent of the women tested HIV positive. The questionnaire showed that 94% of the women knew that sex without condoms could lead to HIV infection, but condoms were only used, on average, in one out of every three acts of sexual intercourse. The results also revealed important knowledge gaps and misconceptions: 68% thought AIDS could be contracted through mosquito bites, and 84% believed that regular blood tests would prevent infection.

After the seminar, the programme tried to persuade the brothel owners to promote the use of condoms among clients; although some agreed to allow the sex workers to refuse a client who would not use a condom, they would not make this an order.

The programme also tried to recruit peer educators from among the sex workers, but this was not successful as the workers changed their workplace frequently and the peer educators claimed they had no authority. Programme staff visited those who tested positive to give support and address their concerns. The constraints faced in this component encouraged programme staff to approach the police to ensure that brothel owners insist on the use of condoms, and to work more aggressively with the younger sex workers.

MOTORCYCLE TAXI DRIVERS

Around 650 men were thought to work as motorcycle taxi drivers in Klong Toey and the sexual behaviour of many of this group put them at high risk of HIV infection. In 1990, the AIDS programme organised two one-day training sessions attended by 498 motorcycle taxi drivers, with an average age of 26. During the session, a survey was conducted to determine each man's age, marital status, sexual behaviours and knowledge of HIV/AIDS. When asked if they frequented brothels, 71% replied that they did so at least once a month, but only 9% reported that they used a condom every time, and over half said they regarded condoms as a nuisance. Only 139 (28%) of the participants took up the offer to have their blood tested for HIV int'ection, and only two of these tested positive: This result was not felt to be representative because most of those practising high-risk behaviour declined to have their blood tested.

Participants in the training sessions were taught about HIV and AIDS, and particularly about the use of condoms. They were encouraged to talk with their clients about AIDS, and given small information cards as memory aides. To encourage discussions, they were also provided with T-shirts and distinctive pink vests carrying AIDS messages. The programme put up billboards with AIDS information at motorcycle taxi stops. A review of the situation some time later found that the motorcycle taxi drivers talked about AIDS only if their clients made comments or asked questions about the slogans on their vest or T-shirt. Either they did not yet have the self-confidence to broach the subject of their own accord, or this was felt to be culturally inappropriate. The programme planned to conduct a follow-up survey of motorcycle taxi drivers to see how much knowledge about HIV/AIDS they had retained. The survey also taught them that to influence condom-use among these young men, who felt they were too young to die, they needed to focus their efforts on explaining the pros and cons of condoms, thus allowing them to make an informed decision.

THE GENERAL PUBLIC

Before Duang Prateep decided on the contents of an AIDS prevention campaign, it carried out a baseline KAP survey among a sample ot residents. The results showed that although 90% of those interviewed knew that AIDS could be contracted through sexual intercourse or sharing needles with an infected person, there were also many alarming misconceptions and knowledge gaps. Half the respondents believed that HIV could be transmitted by mosquitoes, by sneezing, by sharing soap or clothes, or simply by talking with an infected person. Only 33% knew that a person with HIV can still look healthy, and only 34% suggested the use ot condoms as protection against infection. Half thought they could easily be infected simply by sharing a house with an infected person, and only 41% said they would remain friends with a person with AIDS.

The programme's initial response was to mount a series of high-profile public events with the broadest possible mass appeal. The activities included a rally and speeches by prominent persons, AIDS education bulletin boards were erected, posters displayed, and stickers and pamphlets distributed. Over the next several months, similar mass events were organised; a week-long AIDS exhibition, a 'Slogan for AIDS' competition, and a parade through the streets of the neighbourhood.

But the programme staff soon realised that all the activities were attracting the same group of active and interested members of the community; a large proportion of the community was not participating at all. A KAP study carried out seven months atter the launch of the programme found little or no change in either knowledge or in attitudes towards people with HIV/AIDS.

These findings led to a reassessment of the AIDS programme strategy and efforts to improve participation by a number of methods. A small team started to take a mobile audio-visual presentation on AIDS issues to the slum communities, followed up by a question-and-answer session, and this became the focus of community activity. The programme also organised one-day educational seminars for key groups in the community, such as the police, youth leaders, kindergarten parents, women and school students, in the hope that they would become trusted sources of information about AIDS within their families, at their workplace, and with their neighbours and friends. Duang Prateep also decided to broaden their volunteer base. It trained a group of housewives to act as volunteer AIDS educators, visiting their neighbours to teach them about AIDS, and providing regular supplies of free condoms.

The programme planned to expand its activities into nine additional Klong Toey communities and had completed baseline surveys in each area. The surveys would be repeated in the future to evaluate the success of the educational activities. They also planned to increase work with children, to bring prevention into the schools and existing youth groups in the community. Duang Prateep did not plan to provide medical care to people with HIV/AIDS and their families. They felt that other, more specialised agencies were better equipped to provide this service and that their own unique strength lay in their deep roots within and their relationship with, the communities of Klong Toey.

Discussion Questions

1. What strategies did ACT use to try and match its AIDS activities to the needs of the community?
2. To what extent did ACT achieve the objectives of its AIDS programme?
3. What suggestions could you make to ACT on how it might assess the effectiveness of their programme?
4. What recommendations would you make to ACT on the activities and the approaches it might build into its AIDS programme in the future?

THE AIDS COUNSELLING AND TRAINING CENTRE

HOW IT STARTED

The AIDS Counselling and Training (ACT) programme began work in Klong Toey in November 1990. The programme was managed by World Concern International, a US-based Christian organisation with over 10 years experience working with displaced persons and community-based projects in Thailand. Funding was provided by Norwegian Church Aid.

World Concern's original intention was to start an AIDS counselling and testing centre in one of Bangkok's red light districts. On closer examination, however, it became clear that trying to reach commercial sex workers at their workplace would only appear to threaten their livelihood. As one pimp said, "If you even mention the word 'AIDS' around here people will run from you."

After further investigation it was decided to start an AIDS outreach programme in Klong Toey. This decision was influenced by several factors. Klong Toey represented a well-defined community in need of AIDS intervention and community leaders were willing to participate in the kind of project that ACT wanted to put together. ACT knew of no other organisation that was involved in AIDS counselling in the slum communities. The choice was also influenced by the existence of the "Poor People's Clinic", which had been started by a Church organisation but had been forced to close down 12 months earlier due to a lack of operating funds. Renamed the 'ACT Center', the clinic became the operational base for the ACT programme in Klong Toey, while also providing two hours of outpatient medical services five days a week.

THE AIMS OF THE PROGRAMME

The goal of ACT's programme was to prevent HIV infection by educating the community about HIV/AIDS, especially those practising high-risk behaviours. In working with such groups, the programme aimed to promote risk reduction through behaviour modification, above all through encouraging those with multiple sexual partners to use condoms.

The speciffc objectives that ACT defined for its programme were: to establish an AIDS awareness programme for 15 slum communities in Klong Toey; to counsel individuals practising high-risk behaviours in order to stimulate and assist them to modify, minimize or eliminate these behaviours; to offer free and confidential blood tests to all those at risk of HIV infection, in order to promote modification of high-risk behaviours; to identify a professionally-acceptable referral system for HIVpositive persons and those otherwise at risk; and to establish a system for the training of volunteers from universities, churches and other organizations working for AIDS prevention.

PROGRAMME ACTIVITIES AND STAFFING

One of the initial eonstraints that the programme faced was the lack of personnel with the necessary training and experience to work towards the achievement of the objectives.

ACT was unable to find willing volunteers from Klong Toey, so they identified appropriate men and women drawn from university student groups and from churches participating in the ACT programme and trained them as either 'educators' or 'counsellors'.

ACT recognised the importance of these volunteers: "we relied on feedback from the community to monitor our progress. Volunteers helped us to gauge changes in the communities' perception of the epidemic." By April 1992, the programme had seven full-time staff: a manager/counsellor, a medical advisor, an administrator/counsellor, a laboratory technician, a nurse, and two administrative assistants. The programme was assisted by four part-time volunteer counsellors and 12 volunteer community educators. A doctor also worked 2 hours a day at the out-patient clinic.

The programme was implemented through a two-pronged approach: an outpatient clinic at the ACT Center; and an outreach programme within the community. The clinic offered diagnosis and treatment for common diseases, with referral to government hospitals where necessary. Between November 1990 and July 1991 a total of 1,866 patients attended the clinic. The clinic also provided counselling and HIV testing. Counselling took place in a special room on an individual basis. Testing was completely confidential and done only with the informed consent of the client. Before testing, the client was urged to give up any high risk behaviour. The client was told the test result by a counsellor. The clinic also provided printed materials on AIDS and video films were shown continuously in the waiting room, where a 'floating AIDS counsellor' talked informally with people.

The outreach programme, which began in April 1991, became the centre of ACT's educational activities. It aimed to create a healthy awareness of the nature and spread of HIV, and to promote compassionate attitudes towards those already infected with HIV. On Tuesday and Saturday afternoons, trained volunteers carried out house-to-house visits in order to contact, inform, educate and stimulate behaviour change among community members at risk of HIV infection because of high-risk behaviours. The volunteers carried supplies of attractively designed educational materials (a booklet, bookmarks and stickers), which at first glance had no obvious connection with AIDS. This made it easier for people to accept and use the materials. A nurse also accompanied the outreach team to take blood, after on-the-spot counselling, from those wishing to be tested for HIV. The result of the test was communicated to the person at the ACT Center, after further counselling.

A special aspect of the outreach programme consisted of contacting locally-based female sex workers through the owners or managers of the brothels where they lived and worked. ACT made contact with the owners by asking the brothel staff whether the management would allow the young women to receive counselling and voluntary testing. This was done in the spirit of helping them and their employees. Several brothel owners subsequently referred their sex workers for testing at the clinic.*

There was a growing group of NGOs which, though not providing AIDS services, opened their doors to people affected by AIDS in one way or another. World. Concern had begun a forum where Christian organisations met every other month to discuss relevant issues and to coordinate efforts. But although individuals might realise that they needed help, they refused to be referred due to the fear of being 'found out'. Wherever possible, ACT did refer individuals to other organisations, including the House of Hope (a halfway house for recovering drug addicts); House ot' Peace (a home for teenage commercial sex workers); ACET (providing follow-up care t'or PWAs); Christian Outreach (providing a paediatric AIDS programme and orphanage); and to Duang Prateep.

BUILDING ON THE ACHIEVEMENTS

Over the 18 months since they started, ACT had covered a lot of ground in their work with the Klong Toey communities and were proud of their achievements. A report of their progress covering the period trom November 1990 to July 1991 showed that an impressive amount had been achieved in the areas of HIV/AIDS information, education, counselling and testing.

The ACT programme was still at the stage of creating widespread public awareness of the nature and extent of the AIDS epidemic within the Klong Toey neighbourhood. During the next stage, ACT intended to initiate specific activities aimed at reducing the spread of the epidemic and meeting the most urgent needs of HIV-infected individuals and their- families. Strategies they were considering included, t'or example, peer education among high-risk groups such as female prostitutes and injecting drug users, and the training of local volunteers to work with other sections of the community, including people with HIV/AIDS and their families.

THE DUANG PRATEEP FOUNDATION

CASE SYNOPSIS

Discussion Question 1:

What strategies did Duang Prateep use to try and match its HIV/AIDS activities to the needs of the community ?

** An example of the impact of this approach was when the employees of one massage parlour all came together to the clinic for counselling. These young women officially provided massage, but in reality offered sex services as well to earn extrF money. After counselling, they all agreed together that they would no longer provide sex services as this exposed them to the risk of HIV infection.*

EXHIBIT 1

Achievements November 1990 - July 1991

ACTIVITY	VOLUME	COMMENTS/AMPLIFICATION
INFORMATION:		
-Stickers distributed	5,978	
-Booklets distributed	10,573	
-Bookmarks distributed	10,820	
-Clients watching Video	2,976	
EDUCATION:		
- Persons talked to by volunteers	10,203	The total number of persons with whom the volunteers have talked represent 1 in 5 of the adolescent and adult population of Klong Toey. The discussions were conducted either on a one to one basis, in family units or in peer groups. Each session lasted from 5-14 minutes and involved questions and answers. Topics included: HIV and how it is transmitted; the symptoms of AIDS; the implications of having the HIV test; high risk behaviours and ways of modifying or eliminating them. Particular attention was given to dispelling misconceptions about the HIV/AIDS and to the need for care and support within the home for people with AIDS-related illnesses.
COUNSELLING:		
- Pcrsons counselled	3,102	Various types of counselling were carried out by the programme, including: (a) mandatory pre-test counselling, done individually or in groups, either at the ACT Center or in the community. This counselling ensures that clients understand the purpose of the HIV test and the possible implications of the result; (b) discussions about high-risk behaviours, either individually or in groups, to exchange views on how to modify or eliminate them; (c) individual, in-depth counselling in which

		clients examine their own high-risk behaviour and consider safer alternatives; (d) reinforcement counselling, carried out through home visits, for clients who fail to appear at the ACT Center to receive their test result; (e) post-test counselling carried out individually at the ACT Center, regardless of whether the result is positive or negative.
HIV TESTING: - Persons tested (using the Dupont HIV Chek)	621	Positive results were confirmed by Elisa tests carried out by the Thai Red Cross. During this period, a total of persons (7%) tested positive, of whom 30 were identified through the community outreach programme; another 10 were female sex workers referred by brothel owners. Some 93% of those who tested HIV-positive belonged to three groups female sex workers, injecting drug users and male heterosexuals - although these groups accounted for only 45% of those tested. Female spouses accounted for 50% of the tests but only one member of this group tested positive. Unless prevention efforts are effective, however, many more wives are likely to become HIV-positive in the near future.

- Duang Prateep had been working in Klong Toey for 12 years or more, so already had considerable experience and understanding of the problems of the community.
- Most of the staff and volunteers came from Klong Toey, which again helped them to understand the community and its needs.
- The first thing Duang Prateep did after it decided that they had to get involved in AIDS, was to call community leaders together to learn more about HIV/AIDS and to jointly decide on priorities for action.
- Duang Prateep staff held meetings with the sex workers and motorcycle taxi drivers before activities were started.
- Before deciding on any detailed interventions, Duang Prateep conducted surveys of the client groups (IDUs, female sex workers, motorcycle taxi drivers, the general public) to collect data about the lives of the target group, the knowledge, attitudes and practice related to HIV/AIDS, and sexual practices.
- Duang Prateep also carried out subsequent surveys to assess changes in knowledge, attitudes and practices following the intervention or to gain more understanding of what they thought might be important issues (such as the second survey of the IDUs).
- The home visits to the IDUs should also provide some information about what is needed.
- Attempts to get brothel owners to support condom use recognised the power that the brothel owners had over the sex workers and tried to use their influence to contribute to the programme's success.

Discussion Question 2:

How did Duang Prateep assess the effectiveness of its AIDS programme and how were the results of these assessments used to improve its programmes? What suggestions could you make on other ways in which Duang Prateep might evaluate its programmes?

(a) Methods used for assessing effectiveness:

- On the whole, the case suggests that Duang Prateep relied very heavily on surveys of knowledge, attitudes and practice (KAP) to assess the impact of its HIV/AIDS work. Other methods of assessing effectiveness might have helped it to identify intermediate benefits and problems that would assist in programme modification.

- Pre- and post-intervention KAP surveys were carried out. -
- Regular meetings of programme staff were held.
- It can be assumed that Duang Prateep monitored the participation of the sex worker peer group educators in the programme, thus was able to determine that this strategy was not a success.

(b) How the assessments intluenced Duang Prateep's programmes:

- When the idea of trying to get previous IDUs to become peer educators failed, Duang Prateep then decided to use programme staff to carry out the educational activities.
- Data to be collected by Duang Prateep on the age of starting drug use may lead to a new programme focus on children.
- The lack of success in establishing a self-sustaining programme with sex workers has led to an approach to the police to see if they can encourage the brothel owners to insist on condom use by clients.
- The second KAP survey conducted after the mass campaign resulted in a change in approach; namely, the use of a mobile audio-visual presentation, and small group discussion.

(c) Other ways of assessing impact:

Some possible indicators that Duang Prateep might have used include:

- The level and frequency of attendance of IDUs at small group meetings.
- Monitoring the numbers of IDUs who repaid their job-creation loans.
- Monitoring the numbers of IDUs who remained HIV negative.
- Seeking and tracking evidence of self-help/support groups among IDUs and HIV+ persons.
- The number of brothel owner requests for education of their sex workers.

Discussion Question 3:

What recommendations would you make to Duang Prateep on the activities and the approaches they might use in the future as it expands its AIDS programme to a further 9 Klong Toey communities?

- Link up with/coordinate their activities with those of other organisations for referral and further help for clients.
- Make further efforts to try to understand the factors that affect the impact of the programmes with the sex workers and the motorcycle taxi drivers - and may be also the IDUs.
- Search for HIV+ persons willing to "come out" and help in education.
- Start to develop programmes to support those with AIDS and their families.
- Try to link up HIV+ persons with each other so that they can provide mutual support.

THE AIDS COUNSELLING AND TRAINING CENTRE

Discussion Question 1:

What strategies did ACT use to try and match its AIDS activities to the needs of the community?

- Generally, ACT had a difficult time in becoming a "part" of the community. As the case shows, ACT did take a number of steps that helped it to understand what the community needs were and to respond to these through their programme or by referral to others who could help.
- ACT anticipated the problems of HIV/AIDS on the community before this was accepted by the community themselves. This had a significant impact on the programme design and forced ACT to extend its HIV/AIDS activities to include the general health clinic.
- The opening of the clinic was a combination of 'opportunity' and design - the latter because ACT realised that this would be a way of establishing a trusting relationship with the community.
- The community obviously needed health services.
- The volunteers, although from outside the community, seem to be providing feedback on needs to the programme staff to be reflected in the programme's activities.
- The approach to the brothel owners was done in a spirit of cooperation.
- Even though ACT itself could not provide all the support services that might have been needed by those identified as HIV positive and their families, ACT did refer such individuals to other organisations for further support.

Discussion Question 2:

To what extent had ACT achieved the objectives of its AIDS programme?

- Referring to ACT's own objectives (which are listed in the case), these were all stated in terms of outputs (to establish educational programme, to offer blood tests, to offer counselling services, etc.). In this sense, ACT achieved its objectives well (see list of outputs given in the case). However, there is no mention of the impact of the programme on knowledge, attitudes and behaviour; or of any impact on the rate of increase in HIV infection.
- The sex workers (masseuses) who came to ask for information was another indication of success.
- That the brothel owners referred their sex workers to the clinic is another indication of impact.

Discussion Question 3:

What suggestions could you make to ACT on how it might assess the effectiveness of its programme?

- Monitoring the number of individuals coming to the clinic for STD services, for information, and for voluntary HIV testing.
- Monitoring the numbers of condoms distributed.
- Longitudinal studies of those referred to other organisations.
- Some periodic KAP surveys among those coming to the clinic.
- Evidence of peer group activity/support (such as the masseuses coming, en tnasse, to the clinic).
- Collaborating with Duang Prateep on community surveys to gather data, both on programme impact and on strategies for future programme design.

Discussion Question 4:

What recommendations would you make to ACT on the activities and the approaches it might build into its AIDS programme in the future ?

- Efforts to collaborate with Duang Prateep (and with other organisations working with the Klong Toey communities) in volunteer programme, in information exchange, in community needs assessments, etc.
- Perhaps work with the families of those found to be HIV positive, to provide support and counselling.

- Encouragement and support to HIV+ persons and their families to network with others in similar situations.

General Points about the Case:

- ACT is a Christian organisation, which has a strong mission to spread Christianity as well as to provide support and services to the needy. Those reading the case may have strong views on the rights or wrongs of ACT's approach. However, a more fruitful focus for discussion might be the possible strengths and weaknesses of trying to provide both doctrinal and health promotion messages at the same time - particularly in relation to HIV/AIDS prevention.
- ACT's base is in the United States, although it had been working in Thailand for more than 10 years. Participants might wish to explore some of the advantages and disadvantages this might have posed to ACT in Thailand. For example, the degree of freedom that ACT Thailand enjoyed versus the need to work within the policies of the parent organisation; access to funds, expertise, supplies and materials; ownership by the client community of the NGO's programmes and intentions; etc.

6

Klong Toey: Facing Up to AIDS in A Bangkok Slum

The Duang Prateep Foundation and the AIDS Counselling and Training Centre

GLEN WILIAMS
JINNY HUDDART
KAREN MORITA

PART—II

NOTES ON USING THE CASES

1. There are two Cases of organisations working with the Klong Toey communities, together with a general introduction to the area and to the HIV/AIDS situation in Thailand.
2. The cases may be used as a combined package or reviewed independently of each other. The advantage of using the cases together is that readers or participants can compare the ways in which these two NGOs designed and implemented their programmes for the same client community. If only one of the cases is used for participant analysis in the classroom, the other case might usetully be distributed at the end of the discussion so that individuals can later compare the approaches.
3. Based on the options for using these two cases, the materials relating to Klong Toey consist of:

(a) Learning objectives (common to both Cases);
(b) Discussion questions for the combined Cases;
(c) Discussion questions for the Duang Prateep Case;
(d) Discussion questions for the AIDS Counselling and Training Centre Case;
(e) An introduction to AIDS in Thailand and to Klong Toey;
(f) The Duang Prateep Case;
(g) The AIDS Counselling and Training Centre Case;
(h) Facilitators' Notes for the combined cases, and for each Case individually.
Please note that the Discussion Questions for the use of the combined cases are given at the front of the introduction to Klong Toey ("The Setting"). Discussion Questions for use when the cases are considered independently of each other can be found immediately before the relevant case.

4. The discussion questions are intended to help readers to focus on what are considered to be particularly important issues illustrated in the Case. However, the Case may highlight other interesting points and you are encouraged to examine, analyse and discuss these with others.
5. You should review the Objectives and Discussion Questions before turning to the Case itself. After reading the Case carefully, you should then return to the Discussion Questions and prepare your own responses to these, making notes as appropriate, before discussing the case with others.
6. Doing something oneself is the most effective method of learning. Therefore, to get the maximum benefit from the Case, you should prepare your own analysis of the Case before comparing this with points raised in the Facilitators' Notes.
7. There are no right or wrong answers to the Discussion Questions posed. The important issue is the ability to analyse the factors that are influencing the situation and the use of this analysis to draw conclusions about the future.
8. The case is intended to facilitate discussion on important organisational and programmatic issues; it is not intended to demonstrate good or bad practices, nor to evaluate the work of the organisation represented.

Objectives

1. To explore the strategies by which an NGO can reach out into the communities which it is serving to help it design and implement effective AIDS programmes.

2. To identify the constraints and the opportunities that can be faced by NGOs working to reduce the impact of HIV/AIDS, and to explore how these influence future programme design.
3. To examine the ways in which NGOs can assess the impact of their HIV/AIDS activities and use the results of these assessments to improve the effectiveness of their programmes.

Discussion Questions

1. What do you see as the major differences and similarities between the AIDS programmes of Duang Prateep and ACT in terms of:
   (a) the ways in which they planned and designed their programmes?
   (b) the ways in which the two organisations reached out into the communities?
   (c) the ways in which the two organisations assessed the effectiveness of their programmes?
   (d) the constraints faced by the two organisations in implementing their programmes and the steps they took to overcome these?
   (e) any other issues that you consider important in relation to their programmes?
2. What suggestions would you make to each of the organisations on the approaches and the activities they might include in their AIDS programmes in the future?

THE SETTING

Klong Toey is a low-income neighbourhood bordering the docks along the Chao Phraya River, in the southeast corner of Bangkok. In 1992, there were more than 60,000 people living in some 13,500 family units, making Klong Toey the largest of the many illegal squatter settlements which accounted for about 20% of Bangkok's population of 9 million. Offlcially known as a 'slum' (the English word had entered the Thai language), the neighbourhood was divided into 25 sub-communities, each with an elected council recognised to some extent by the municipal authorities.

The slum dwellers had lived for over 30 years in any left-over, unoccupied land. Many of them had been evicted several times and forced to find another corner of free land, or a shelter along railway tracks or under expressways. Most of the houses were built on stilts above swampland and could be reached only by rickety boardwalks. Basic services such as sanitation and refuse collection were grossly inadequate. Electricity had reached into most of the houses, but water had to be carried in and stored in jars.

Most of the residents had regular, but poorly-paid jobs. Surveys carried out in the 1980s showed that 33% were labourers (in the docks or construction sites), 34% were factory or transport workers, and 10% were traders and food vendors. Literacy rates among the residents were low. Apart from their obvious economic and environmental problems, many of Klong Toey residents had a poor image of themselves as second-class citizens, with little hope of improving their situation.

AIDS AND KLONG TOEY

By 1992, AIDS had become a crisis in Thailand. Over the 4 years from 1988 to 1991, the estimated number of AIDS cases equalled that found in America which had been struggling with the infection for 10 years and had four times the number of citizens. Recent data from Thailand indicated that the national HIV prevalence rate for female sex workers was between 10% and 20%, with a corresponding figure of 32% for injecting drug users. A nationwide survey of 26,000 men between the ages of 20-22 years old found a 2% seropositive rate, with the rate reaching as high as 11 % in the northern provinces.

Certain practices in Thailand are very conducive to the spread of HIV. Commercial sex, although illegal, is popular and widely accepted. It has been estimated that 90% of all Thai men visit a sex worker before the age of nineteen. Surveys conducted in the Klong Toey communities found that 82% of men and 66% of women felt it was normal for men to go to sex workers. Another 76% of men and 83% of women felt that there was nothing wrong with a poor woman becoming a sex worker. At the same time, migration to the cities and the often lucrative nature of commercial sex work helped the expansion of the sex industry. Even in 1992, the use of condoms was not widespread; most men believed that condoms reduced their pleasure and were an insult to their manhood. Drug abuse also remained a serious problem in Thailand and there were large numbers of intravenous heroin users, both in the northern provinces and increasingly in all urban centres.

No surveys of the extent of infection in Klong Toey as a whole had been carried out, but by 1992 it was likely that at least 3% of the total population was already HIV positive. The Klong Toey community included a high proportion of sexually active young people, many injecting drug users (IDUs), and significant numbers of both male and female sex workers and their clients. Among those practising high risk behaviours, the level of infection had been found to be much higher. Despite national and local AIDS campaigns, it had been difficult to impress on the people of Klong Toey the dangers of HIV infection. This was partly due to the long incubation period of the disease. Very few people in Klong Toey had yet developed

AIDS and it was difficult to convince the community of the seriousness of an infection that they could neither see nor feel.

AIDS is expected to affect the lives of a growing number of people in Klong Toey during the mid 1990's, when many HIV-positive IDUs will start showing symptoms. By 1998, an even larger group, including sex workers and their clients, will need medical attention. The burden of providing care for people with AIDS will fall mainly on other family members, especially on women, who are already struggling for survival. A growing number of 'AIDS orphans' - not only HIV-pesitive babies and toddlers but also their non-infected elder siblings - will require care and support. These developments are likely to subject the traditional support system of the Thai extended family to intolerable pressures and strains.

FACILITATORS' NOTES

GENERAL POINTS ABOUT USING THE CASES

1. The materials relating to Klong Toey consist of two cases (the Duang Prateep Foundation and the AIDS Counselling and Training Centre), together with a general introduction to Klong Toey and the AIDS situation in Thailand.
   The cases can be used either separately or together, although this is a lot of reading for the participants. The advantage of discussing them both is that the participants can see the differences in the ways in which the two organisations determined community needs, designed and implemented their programmes, and assessed the impact of their activities. If only one of the cases is to be discussed, it should be accompanied by the general introduction to Klong Toey and AIDS in Thailand. If one case is used in the classroom, the other might usefully be handed out for individual reading at the end of the discussion.

2. Based on the options for using these two cases, three sets of discussion questions and facilitators' notes have been provided: (a) for analysis of the Duang Prateep programme alone; (b) for analysis of the ACT programme alone; (c) for a combined analysis of the two cases.

3. Participants should be encouraged to read the materials and to prepare their own analyses before the classroom discussion. The appropriate discussion questions should be handed out with the cases to assist participants in their analysis.

4. Discussion of either a single or the joint cases is likely to require 1½ to 2 hours (assuming that participants have previously read the case and prepared their own analysis).

5. The discussion questions are intended to help participants to focus on what were considered to be particularly important issues illustrated in the case. However, the case may raise many other interesting points for participants and they should be encouraged to examine, analyse and discuss these if raised.

6. The notes that follow are intended to assist the facilitator to prepare to teach the case. They provide a synopsis of the information given in the case, together with some ideas on strategies that the organisations might consider in the future. These notes should not replace the facilitator's own preparation and analysis. During the discussion, the facilitator's role is to help participants to reach their own conclusions, based upon a thorough analysis of the information given.

7. When introducing participants to the case, the facilitator should stress that the case is intended to facilitate discussion on important organisational and programmatic issues; it is not intended to demonstrate good or bad practices, nor to evaluate the work of the organisations represented.

THE COMBINED CASES: DUANG PRATEEP & THE AIDS COUNSELLING AND TRAINING CENTRE

Discussion Question 1:

What do you see as the major differences and similarities between the AIDS programmes of Duang Prateep and ACT in terms of:

(a) the ways in which they planned and designed their programmes,
(b) the ways in which the two organisations have reached out into the communities;
(c) the ways in which the two organisations have assessed the effectiveness of their programmes,
(d) the constraints faced by the two organisations in implementing their programmes and the steps they have taken to overcome these,
(e) any other issues that you consider important in relation to their programmes.

(a) Programme planning and design:

- Duang Prateep already had experience with and the trust of the community before they began working in the tield of HIV/AIDS prevention; ACT was an externally-based organisation with no previous background in Klong Toey.

- As soon as Duang Prateep decided that it should be concerned about HIV/AIDS, it involved the community in meetings to jointly learn about the epidemic and to begin to identify the needs within Klong Toey. ACT came to Klong Toey with its own agenda. However, both organisations ended up with similar objectives.

- Duang Prateep's background with the community, based on the perceived success of their other social service programs, allowed it to focus immediately on interventions related to HIV/AIDS. Given the sensitive nature of HIV/AIDS, together with some level of denial that it was even a problem for Klong Toey residents, ACT felt it first had to build an entry to the community through the clinic.

- Duang Prateep was clearly experienced in carrying out surveys and used these as means of learning about the groups it had targetted for attention; ACT simply started offering medical services, piggybacking HIV/AIDS counselling, intormation and testing on to these.

(b) Reach into the community:

- Both organisations used volunteers: Duang Prateep used mainly Klong Toey residents; ACT had to search for volunteers outside of Klong Toey due to its lack of relationship with the Klong Toey communities.

- Duang Prateep's roots in Klong Toey allowed it immediate access; ACT had to work slowly to build up trust through the clinic.

- Duang Prateep had targetted specific groups and its staff went out to learn and interact with them. ACT's programme was not specifically targetted at any one group; rather the programme aimed at providing services to the general community (except for their approach to the brothels).

(c) Assessing the effectiveness of the programmes:

- Duang Prateep regularly checked changes in community knowledge, attitudes and practice through surveys; ACT tended to count outputs as a measure of effectiveness.

- ACT set itself clear output objectives; Duang Prateep's objectives were vaguer, although they did try to deal with impact.

- Duang Prateep used regular assessments to change programme strategies; there is no information in the case which indicates that ACT did the same.

(d) Constraints:

- Duang Prateep seemed to have a difficult time in making an impact in any of their programmes, but the staff kept searching for new ways to influence the situation.

- Duang Prateep changed its approach several times (from mass campaign to small group presentations and discussions; from ex-IDUs as peer educators to Duang Prateep volunteers; from promoting condom use at all times among motorcycle taxi drivers to providing them with the information upon which they can make an informed decision for themselves).

- ACT's major constraint was legitimacy - but this appeared to be growing with the clinic's contribution.

- A major constraint for both organisations was that it was difficult to measure whether either of them were achieving their goals of HIV prevention.

(e) Other Issues:

- ACT is a Christian organisation, which has a strong mission to spread Christianity as well as to provide support- and services to the needy. Those reading the case may have strong views on the rights or wrongs of ACT's approach. However, a more fruitful focus for discussion might be the possible strengths and weaknesses of trying to provide both doctrinal and health promotion messages at the same time - particularly in relation to HIV/AIDS prevention.

- ACT is a U.S.based organisation, although it had been working in Thailand for more than 10 years. Duang Prateep was clearly 'owned' by the Klong Toey communities. Participants might wish to explore some of the advantages and disadvantages of these two situations as related to, for example: the degree of freedom that an international NGO enjoys locally versus the need to work within the policies of the parent organisation; access to funds, expertise, supplies and materials; perceptions of the client community of the NGO's programmes and intentions; etc.

- There is little mention in the cases of the relationship, if any, of these NGOs to Government programmes or policies. Participants might wish to discuss the ways in which the Government could support NGO initiatives in HIV/AIDS prevention.

- Participants have been guided to consider the differences between the approaches of the two NGOs as described in the cases, and to suggest ways in which these NGOs might collaborate. It might also be useful for participants to reflect on some of the barriers to such collaboration and strategies that could be used to overcome these where collaboration would clearly benefit the clients. For example: the time it takes; possible differences in organisational philosophy and programme objectives; competition for funds or other resources; etc.

Discussion Question 2:

What suggestions would you make to each of the organisations on the approaches and the activities they might include in their AIDS programmes in the future ?

Duang Prateep:

- Link up with other organisations for the referral of clients who need further or specialised help, support or care.
- Make further efforts to try to understand the constraints affecting the impact of the programmes with the sex workers and the motorcycle taxi drivers - and may be also the IDUs.
- Try to identify HIV+ persons willing to "come out" and help in education among the communities.
- Consider the development of programmes to support persons with AIDS (PWAs) and their families.
- Try to link up HIV+ persons so that they can provide support to each other.
- Seek ways of collaborating with ACT or with other organisations working with the Klong Toey communities. For example, in relation to ACT: referral of individuals to clinic; use of clinic counselling services; sharing of information and experience on successful strategies; collaboration on community KAP or other surveys; approaching ACT to provide information and maybe training for Duang Prateep's volunteers on the importance of the general health of HIV+ individuals and those with AIDS, on STD identification and the importance of treatment, etc.

ACT:

- Consider collaboration with Duang Prateep - in volunteer programme; in information exchange; in community needs assessments; accepting client referrals for counselling, testing and services; training of Duang Prateep statff in such areas as the importance of identifying and treating STDs, etc.

- Possibility of offering outreach support (counselling and/or services) to the families of HIV+ individuals and PWAs.

- Try to encourage and support networking among HIV+ persons and their families.

7

Community Development and AIDS Prevention

The South India AIDS Action Programme, Madras

JENNY HUDDART
CATHERINE OVERHOLT

1. In addition to these notes, the materials relating to the South India AIDS Action Programme consist of:
   - (a) Learning Objectives;
   - (b) Discussion Questions;
   - (c) Thre Case;
   - (d) Facilitators' Notes
2. The discussion questions are intended to help readers to focus on what are considered to be particularly important issues illustrated in the Case. However, the Case may highlight other interesting points and you are encouraged to examine, analyse and discuss these with others.
3. You should review the Objectives and Discussion Questions before turning to the Case itself. After reading the Case carefully, you should then return to the Discussion Questions and prepare your own responses to these, making notes as appropriate, before discussing the case with others.

4. Doing something oneself'is the most effective method of learning. Therefore, to get the maximum benefit from the Case, you should prepare your own analysis of the Case before comparing this with points raised in the Facilitators' Notes.
5. There are no right or wrong answers to the Discussion Questions posed. The important issue is the ability to analyse the factors that are influencing the situation and the use of this analysis to draw conclusions about the future.
6. The case is intended to facilitate discussion on important organisational and programmatic issues; it is not intended to demonstrate good or bad practices, nor to evaluate the work of the organisation represented.

Objectives

1. To develop participants' understanding of the organisational issues that may be faced by a newly-established NGO as it tries to respond to the demands for HIV/AIDS interventions.
2. To identify and evaluate the strategies that can be used to maintain organisational effectiveness.
3. To examine the implications of relying on external funding for programme sustainability and to identify strategies which an NGO can use to develop support from local sources.

Discussion Questions

1. What strategies did SIAAP use to identify community needs for HIV/AIDS interventions and to determine SIAAP's response? What are the advantages and disadvantages of the approach it took?
2. What do you see as the possible organisational problems that may face SIAAP within the next 12 months? What suggestions could you make to help SIAAP deal with these?
3. What impact did donor funding have on SIAAP? What steps could SIAAP take to minimise the disadvantages of external funding? What strategies might SIAAP use to further develop the support it gets from local sources?
4. What recommendations would you make to Shyamla and the SIAAP team on how they might continue to develop their programmes in the future?

"We've just had our first State level workshop, for NGOs working in Tamil Nadu State. Around 45 NGOs were represented at the workshop, all of whom had expressed their interest in developing interventions related to HIV/AIDS to complement their existing programmes. With help from experienced resource people from across the country, the workshop focused on the components of effective interventions, how to go about programme design, and how to look for funding. It was really hard, especially dealing with all the administrative arrangements. The whole SIAAP team had to drop their other work to help me organise the workshop. Our efforts paid off; after all the many months of preparation in the Districts, the workshop was very successful. Now we have to start preparing for the next State workshop to be held in Hyderabad later this year."

HOW IT ALL STARTED

In 1988, the PANOS Institute in England commissioned Shyamla, then an independent journalist with little interest or knowledge of AIDS, to write the story of a group of women, diagnosed as HIV positive, who were detained in the Vigilance Home in Madras.

Because of official fears of publicity, it took Shyamla six months to gain access to the women, and when eventually she did, it was a very emotional and shocking experience. Unable to drop the matter, and after getting legal advice, Shyamla decided to take the matter to the courts, bringing a case against the Government for unlawful detention. Shyamla won the case and the women were released from detention in July 1990. While the case was still being contested, Shyamla travelled around India researching follow-up articles for PANOS on the availability of support services in relation to HIV/AIDS. She found none. She began to realise that advocacy alone is of little use without a supporting infrastructure and she was haunted by the question of what would happen to the women upon their release. The idea that she wanted to "help set up support systems in a society that was so obviously unprepared and as obviously bound to need them sooner or later" was born.

In November 1990, Shyamla attended an international seminar in Paris for NGO's working in HIV/AIDS and was struck by the lack of examples of HIV/AIDS programmes that had been integrated into existing community development work. She was convinced that such integration was vital in India and discussed her ideas with the other participants. As a direct result, she was offered $30,000 from the WHO Partnership programme to implement three State-level NGO workshops to promote their development of HIV/AIDS activities. The PANOS Institute in London was to be the international partner.

On her return to Madras, Shyamla searched for an appropriate organisational home for the project, but found that NGOs at that time were not interested in AIDS. Realising that she would have to move ahead on her own, Shyamla used personal contacts to establish a link with the Voluntary Health Services, which agreed to provide her with a project account for the channelling of funds and to rent her an office, at a nominal charge to cover utility costs.

To launch the project and to get help in accessing NGOs in Tamil Nadu, Shyamla contacted existing NGO networks. The Chairwoman of one of these, the State Social Welfare Board, provided indispensable help. She offered to call meetings of the voluntary agencies in each of the Districts if Shyarnla would take responsibility for the agenda and content. Shyamla accepted the challenge and, although no project funds had yet arrived, went ahead with the first workshop in February, 1991. The workshop informed the NGOs about HIV/AIDS and discussed the likely impact of the epidemic on the communities with which they were working. The NGOs showed considerable interest and Shyamla was looking forward to the next District workshop.

As expenses mounted Shyamla was well aware that she could not continue indefinitely to count on the generosity of her family and friends to advance funds to the project. Then, PANOS informed her that the WHO contribution would be less than anticipated. By this time, the workshops were scheduled with the Districts, materials were being designed and printed, and Shyamla was concerned that her own professional reputation would suffer if the project came to an abrupt halt. In desperation, she contacted the Ford Foundation, which had also been represented at the Paris seminar. To her great relief, it agreed to support the project and the first financial installment arrived in September, 1991. (See Exhibit 2.) By then, Shyamla had already completed ten district workshops, with more than 200 NGOs attending. She had developed and distributed a calendar and information booklets, and had informed participating NGOs that those who were interested in developing HIV/AIDS programmes should contact SIAAP and formally request an invitation to the State workshop which was to be held early in 1992. In October 1991, the Partnership Programme was also able to release US$15,000 for SIAAP to the PANOS institute.

SIAAP AND ITS PROGRAMMES

Organisation and Staffing

By early 1992, there were seven staff working with SIAAP. (See Exhibit 1.) SIAAP was soon to lose Nandini, who would be getting married and following her husband to Bombay. A second member, Roma, was also scheduled to leave Madras in 1993, to join her husband at his new military posting. Recognising that they needed to make more formal arrangements for the accounts, the SIAAP team had begun the search for a part-time accountant to help them maintain their financial records and produce their financial reports. The volume of correspondence and documentation passing through the office was also forcing them to think of getting computer-literate secretarial help.

The single-room office had become far too cramped and the team was looking for larger office space and a sponsor to pay the rent. In May 1992, SIAAP was to become a registered voluntary organisation, with the right to maintain its own funds, rather than having them channelled through an intermediary such as VHS or PANOS. The original project funding was to end in October 1992.

The NGO Support Programme

The District workshops revealed that NGOs would need considerable help to implement HIV/AIDS intervention programmes. Although the NGOs had agreed that sexually-transmitted diseases (STDs) were a common problem in their communities, they said they were unable either to talk about them or to provide or link up with any kind of diagnostic and clinical services. Condom promotion was rare, with most NGOs focusing on types of family planning methods for which women take responsibility. Few NGOs had any experience in collecting and analysing information to help assess programme needs. Many had difficulty in identitying possible intervention strategies tor STD/HIV prevention, tending to stick to approaches with which they were already familiar. Programme monitoring and evaluation were almost non-existent. Most importantly, in relation to HIV/AIDS, the staff was unaccustomed to talking to their clients about sex and sexuality and needed help in developing communication skills in this area.

SIAAP was given its first opportunity to provide follow-up support to an NGO when in April 1991 the Madras Christian Council of Social Services (MCCSS) asked for help in setting up an AIDS education programme in the slums where it was working. Shyamla helped MCCSS to design and conduct a survey to assess the needs of the slum communities, to develop an appropriate intervention strategy and programme, and to recruit and train programme staff. It soon became clear that in order to effectively integrate the AIDS programme into the work of the organisation, all the MCCSS staff needed information and training on HIV/AIDS. Shyamla also worked with staff to help them overcome their reluctance to talk about sex and to encourage nonjudgemental attitudes. As Shyamla said, "the MCCSS staff changed from a group that did not use the word 'sex' if a substitute could be found, to a situation where condom jokes were heard freely around the office". This work with MCCSS was very valuable for Shyamla, giving her the chance to actually experience what SIAAP was asking other NGOs to do. It also confirmed for Shyamla that SIAAP had an important role to play as a resource for other NGOs and convinced her that SIAAP should continue to be involved in programme implementation if they were to be able to help other NGOs to do the same.

Other SIAAP Programmes

By keeping the project workshop costs to a minimum, by volunteering their time wherever possible, and by seeking local sponsorship, the SIAAP team managed to stretch the project funds over a number of other activities. These activities were in line with SIAAP's intention to develop model HIV/AIDS interventions that could provide examples to, and be replicated by, other NGOs.

The lorry drivers' health education programme was started by Kumar in October, 1991. His previous experience had shown that simply giving out STD information and condoms had little effect on behaviour, so this programme started with a survey of 200 lorry drivers at a check post some 30 kms. outside of Madras. The results of the survey showed that almost 90% of the drivers had visited commercial sex workers, more than 90% had had some torm of STD, but less than 30% regularly used condoms. The drivers said that they would welcome somewhere to relax at the checkpoint as well as information about STDs and AIDS. In response, Kumar set up a health education booth at the check point where the drivers could relax and get entertaining STD/AIDS information, including details of where to go for treatment, and obtain condoms of different makes. By April 1992, there were indications that the programme had had some impact. The lorry drivers were asking more questions about STDs, were requesting more condoms, and had asked for STD services to be provided at the checkpoint. In addition, a number of other NGOs, who had learned about the programme at the State workshop, had asked SIAAP to help them replicate it at other check points.

Nandini's previous experience had led to the design and implemention of a training programme for volunteers in Madras. The programme, run jointly with Kate, trained individuals to become peer educators for HIV prevention in their communities. Training in telephone counselling was to be included in the programme in the near future. With the help of these volunteers, SIAAP had already mounted puppet shows and street theatre, using traditional folk media, to help communicate the HIV/AIDS prevention messages to the urban slum communities with whom MCCSS was working.

Roma's training and experience helped her to conduct a study of the Mauras slum dwellers' access to services for sexually transmitted diseases (STDs). It was estimated that one out of every 20 people in India suffered from an STD, and there were many reports from the slum women of infertility, frequent miscarriage and leucorrhoea (all indications of potential STDs). The study showed that whilst men were well aware of the dangers of STDs and sought medical attention (and penicillin shots) after "risky" sex, women would seek treatment only if they had an obvious problem. Women also tended to use private practitioners. Use of Government services by women was low, largely due to the lack of female specialists, the lack of STD services in the nearby clinics, the absence of adequate privacy, the judgemental attitudes of the doctors and the costs of travelling to the hospital. NGOs working in the slum areas tended to focus on basic MCH services and referred any STD problems to the general hospital. The report indicated an urgent need for STD services to be provided in the slums, preferably a mobile clinic that could cover a larger catchment area. Roma found out that the Ministry of Health already had a van equipped to provide STD services, but lacked a female STD specialist or gynaecologist to run it. Over the next year, Roma planned to focus on finding ways to meet some of the STD needs identified by the survey.

THE FUTURE

The SIAAP members bubbled with ideas for the future. A priority for them was to start an HIV/AIDS "hotline", a telephone service, aimed at the urban community of Madras, to answer queries and provide a supportive ear to callers. A sponsor for the first year of the hotline service had been found, and SIAAP needed to train their own staff and volunteers in counselling to be able to answer the calls.

Another exciting opportunity had also arisen. SIAAP had contracted with a private market research company to design and implement a KAP survey in one of the Districts. This company subsequently approached SIAAP to suggest that they would be willing, at their own expense, to document their experience in the form of a manual which could then be used to guide others through the process. They were also willing to train SIAAP staff in the methodology so that, in turn, SIAAP members could support other NGOs. SIAAP needed to find the time to work with this company on the development of the manual .

Shyamla was adamant that SIAAP's mission was to be a resource centre for NGOs for the development of integrated community development and HIV/AIDS programmes. SIAAP should be able to provide these NGOs with information, training, technical support and materials. SIAAP should also help to create and sustain networks among these NGOs so that they can learn from each others' experiences and support each other. On the other hand, the team felt strongly that SIAAP should take advantage of the considerable skills and experience of the team members to design and implement its own programmes as model interventions.

Another principle that the team members felt very strongly about related to how SIAAP activities should be funded. While they appreciated the invaluable contributions that had been made by "outsiders", their ideal was for all SIAAP activities to be financed trom local sources - including donations of people's time, materials and funds from Indian organisations and individuals, and contributions from the beneficiaries (communities) themselves.

The team believed that true development (and this included dealing with HIV/AIDS) could only be achieved by self-supported and self-sustaining action. The team members recognised that this might not always be possible as the HIV epidemic will not wait for development; but they were haunted by the image of being dependent upon, and even under the control of, external donors.

The SIAAP members were a very close team who knew and worked with each other well. They derived great satisfaction and learned a lot from talking about their work and ideas with each other. By April 1992, they had begun to feel the pressure of the rapidly-increasing volume of work and knew that the demands on SIAAP were likely to grow as more and more NGOs became active in HIV/AIDS. Shyamla had already confessed to "being consumed" by the work - meaning both her own drive and commitment to what SIAAP was trying to achieve, and the sheer lack of time she had available to devote to anything else.

In the meantime, SIAAP was planning another State-level workshop for September 1992.

Facilitator's Notes

GENERAL POINTS ABOUT USING THE CASE

1. Participants should be encouraged to read the case and to prepare their own analysis before it is discussed with others in the classroom. The discussion questions should be handed out with the case to assist participants in their analysis.

2. Generally, discussion of this case has required 1½ to 2 hours (assuming that participants have previously read the case and prepared their own analysis).

3. The discussion questions included with this case are intended to help participants to focus on what were considered to be particularly important issues illustrated in the case. However, the case may raise many other interesting points for participants and they should be encouraged to examine, analyse and discuss these if raised.

COMMUNITY DEVELOPMENT AND AIDS PREVENTION
The South India AIDS Action Programme, Madras

EXHIBIT 1
Siaap Staff In March 1992

NAME	POS ITION	PREVIOUS EXPERIENC E	SIAAP RESPONSIBILITIES
Shyamla Nataraj	SIAAP Coordinator	Independent journalist, with a Masters' Degree in Communication. Founder of SIAAP.	Overall responsibility for SIAAP programmes and staff. Primary responsibility for the NGO Support programme and for SIAAP's financial management.
G. Kı aresan (Kumar)	Programme Officer	Masters' Degree in Social Work. Previously worked on another Madras AIDS project. assisting with the implementation of a health education programme for lorry drivers .	Responsible for the design and implementation of SIAAP's Lorry Drivers Education Programme. Now seeking to expand the programme to other check points and to assist other NGOs in replicating the model developed by SIAAP.
Nandini Rao	Programme officer	Masters Degree in French, obtained in the USA. Whilst studying in the US, she worked as a volunteer on an AIDS programme in Pennsylvania.	Responsible for the design and implementation of SIAAP's volunteer training programme.
Roma Soloman	Programme officer	A qualified doctor, with many years of experience in community-based health programmes, panicularly those dealing with leprosy and STDs.	Responsible for the promotion of STD services for women living in the Madras slums.

NAME	POS ITION	PREVIOUS EXPERIENC E	SIAAP RESPONSIBILITIES
Babur Sheriff	Health Educator	Studying for his degree in Social Work	Assists Kumar in the Lorry Driver Education Programme.
V. Premaja	Office Administrator	MA and MPhil in public administration. Strong interest in womens' involvement in the economy and industry.	Responsible for organising SIAAP's office library and for administrative tasks.
Kate Shechter	Volunteer	Conducting her PhD research in anthropology on the religious responses to AIDS in India. An American national AIDS activist and feminist.	Assists, as required, on all of SIAAP's programmes. In particular, responsible for working with Nandini on the volunteer training programme.

4. The notes that follow are intended to assist the facilitator to prepare to teach the case. They provide a synopsis of the information given in the case, together with some ideas on strategies that SIAAP might adopt in the future. These notes should not replace the facilitator's own preparation and analysis. At all times, the facilitator should encourage the participants to reach their own conclusions, based upon a thorough analysis of the information given.

5. When introducing participants to the case, the facilitator should stress that the case is intended to facilitate discussion on important organisational and programmatic issues; it is not intended to demonstrate good or bad practices, nor to evaluate the work of SIAAP.

CASE SYNOPSIS

Discussion Question 1:

What strategies did SIAAP use to identify community needs for HIV/AIDS interventions and to determine SIAAP's response? What are the advantages and disadvantages of the approach it took?

(a) Strategies Used to Identify Community Needs:

- Informal research. Shyamla's initial experience with the women detained at the Vigilance Home and her subsequent research into support mechanisms for HIV+ individuals and persons with AIDS (PWAs) provided clear evidence of the lack of services and resources in the communities.

- Especially-designed needs assessments: (i) Shyamla's assistance to MCCSS for the development of HIV/AIDS interventions started with her helping them to design and conduct a survey of community needs within the selected slum areas. It is assumed that MCCSS had previous knowledge and understanding of the overall development needs of the communities through their existing programmes. (ii) The lorry drivers' education programme started with a survey of the situation and the wishes of the lorry drivers themselves. (iii) Suspicions of the situation regarding STDs in the slum areas of Madras prompted a full-scale field investigation of the situation and the needs of the women before any assumptions were made about appropriate interventions.

- The District KAP survey (presumably conducted to help another NGO to design appropriate HIV prevention interventions).

- The information gathered during the first NGO workshop, which helped SIAAP to identify the experience and support needs of the NGOs. The District workshops also provided Shyamla with information regarding the existing programmes of community-based organisations and helped her to identify the strengths and weaknesses of these organisations in relation to implementing HIV/AIDS interventions. Shyamla then encouraged the NGOs to get back to her if they were interested in getting further support for implementation of projects (i.e. to define their needs first).
- Evidence of any needs assessment in the case of the volunteer training programme or the hotline is not available. From the information given in the case, these appear to have grown out of the specific interests of individual members of the SIAAP team. On the other hand, it would be difficult in these instances to determine community needs for these programmes, particularly if no similar programmes already exist in the locality.

(b) Strategies Used to Determine SIAAP's Response:

- Initially, Shyamla awarded priority to supporting other, existing community development NGOs to develop their own HIV/AIDS programmes. However, each new person joining SIAAP seems to have started his or her own activities, based on individual professional interests and previous experience. Although all efforts to stem HIV infection rates are needed, SIAAP's situation could result in a lack of focus, the diversion of efforts away from priority areas and an over-extension of the NGO and its staff. On the other hand, the commitment and motivation of the individual SIAAP members are essential to the survival and effectiveness of the organisation.
- Participants should be asked to consider how a balance might be achieved between 'rational decision-making' about work priorities and allowing the individual members (some of whom are unpaid volunteers) sufficient freedom to pursue areas they feel to be important.
- The information given in the case suggests that SIAAP has given more attention to identifying the needs for HIV/AIDS interventions than to considering whether SIAAP really has the resources to respond effectively to those needs. Participants might be asked to identify the factors that an NGO needs to consider when making a decision on what activities it should or should not initiate.

(c) Advantages/Disadvantages of the Approach Taken:

Possible advantages include: (i) the design and implementation of intervention programs provided SIAAP with direct experience in the field and. kept them in touch with both community needs and the programmes of other NGOs; (ii) SIAAP's direct field experience would have increased their credibility with other NGOs, thus facilitating the acceptance of their guidance and support; (iii) the intervention programmes allowed staff to pursue their interests and the field work provided them with direct feedback from clients; both of which may have helped to maintain the members' commitment and motivation; (iv) SIAAP's programmes provided "demonstration" sites which would be of help in the 'training' of less-experienced NGOs; (v) by implementing field programmes, SIAAP provided much-needed services to the community; (vi) some potential donors might have been more interested in supporting field interventions than funding SIAAP's NGO support programme.

Possible disadvantages include: (i) confusion over SIAAP's priorities; (ii) excessive work demands on staff and/or volunteers; (iii) over-extension of the staff and the organisation; (iii) possible lack of continuity in programmes (intervention programmes may terminate abrüptly if the responsible SIAAP member leaves the organisation).

Discussion Questiion 2:

What do you see as the possible organisational (internal) problems that may face SIAAP within the next 12 months? What suggestions could you make to help SIAAP deal with these?

(a) Organisational Mission/Programme Focus:

Possible problems include: (i) confusion over priorities (for example, all SIAAP staff had to drop their programme work to help Shyamla organise the State level workshop); (ii) conflict within the individual team members between 'doing the work themselves' as against helping others to implement programmes; (iii) inability to respond to NGO requests for help due to an overload of work on SIAAP staff and/or volunteers; (iv) division of staff into "doers" and "helpers of other NGOs", with the potential for one group's work being viewed as less important; (v) SIAAP's own model interventions could blind them to the potential of other models proposed or pursued by other NGOs.

Possible strategies include: (i) establishment of clear priorities, discussed with all staff and volunteers; (ii) development and agreement of clear criteria for SIAAP's involvement in direct implementation. Such criteria could include the sort of interventions that SIAAP should implement, the duration of such programmes, their purpose, how they will be handed over to others for continuation/replication, the number of interventions at any one time, etc.; (iii) the development of an annual workplan with the statf, establishing targets and/or limits on the numbers and kinds of interventions that can be implemented, taking into account both the projected workload involved with maintaining an adequate NGO support programme, and overall statting/funding limitations; (iv) at the time of recruitment, SIAAP's priorities and limitations could be made clear to new staff members or volunteers; (v) if statf are very keen to get directly involved in programme interventions, SIAAP might search for ways of enabling them to do this by participating in another organisation's programmes. (i.e. secondments);

(b) Workload

Possible problems include: (i) dit'ficulty in maintaining programme focus; (ii) over-commitment of staff in trying to meet demands; (iii) inability to meet support needs of NGOs; (iv) conflict where staff member doesn't have the same "all consuming" commitment as leader.

Possible strategies include: regular review and rein for cement of SIAAP's mission with staff and volunteers; (ii) review of the implications of each proposed activity before taking the decision to implement; (iii) establishment of clear priorities among the activities and responsibilities of both the organisation and the individual staff members and volunteers; (iv) monitoring the workload of staff and volunteers; (v) regular review of the organisation and the programmes; (vi) recognition that the time each individual can ot't'er to SIAAP is based on personal circumstances.

(c) Staffing:

Possible problems include: (i) conflict between salaried staff and volunteers; (ii) when SIAAP's 'pathfinder' role turns into a 'maintenance' role. the organisation may lose the interest of the leader and founding members; (iii) the demands placed on the organisation may put pressure on SIAAP to expand too fast; (iv) it could be difficulties to maintain the initial enthusiasm exhibited by the initial team as new people join SIAAP; (v) the difficulties of assimilating new members into the team.

Potential strategies include: (i) SIAAP could deliberately seek to recruit members whose strengths and interests lie in program maintenance rather than 'breaking new ground"; (ii) defining clear criteria for the recruitment of new members; (iii) open discussion about the fact that volunteering one's time (as opposed to being paid a salary) is a personal decision; (iv) conscious efforts may need to be made to help new members feel equally important to the finding members of the team.

(d) Funding:

Possible problems include: (i) the pressure to implement programmes could overwhelm caution in relation to external funding; (ii) the problem of paying the salaries for additional staff; (iii) continued uncertainty over funding sources and levels, making it difficult to plan or attract staff.

Possible strategies include: (i) establishing criteria for acceptance of donor funding; (ii) allocating responsibility for fund raising to a specific individual or individuals; (iii) considering the question of financial sustainability at the time of making workplan decisions; (iv) SIAAP might use its NGO networks to help identify potential funding sources for its activities.

(e) Administration:

Possible problems include: (i) as SIAAP grows, there will be increasing need to develop more formal administrative procedures for financial management and accounting, work planning, recruitment and allocation of work, etc.; (ii) there may be difficulties in finding office space and a reliable sponsor to cover the rent; (iii) the administrative burden on the leader will increase and she may find that more of her time is taken up with administration, thus detracting from her ability to remain closely involved in all the programme activities. This may also reduce her enjoyment of the work.

Possible strategies include: (i) assessing each new administrative system to ensure that it is essential, and that it achieves the objective in the simplest way possible; (ii) regular review of administrative systems to ensure that they remain subordinate to programme goals; (iii) ensuring that administrative staff and their allocated responsibilities are guided by programme needs; (iv) involving all staff in discussions of administrative issues to help prevent the administration becoming an end in itself; (v) as far as possible, giving all staff some administrative responsibilities, so that the divide between administrative and programme staff is kept to a minimum.

(f) Work planning and coordination:

Possible problems include: (i) growth may bring increasing difficulties in coordinating activities; (ii) with more members it will become more difficult to share experiences; (iii) with growth, there will be greater need to establish clear work priorities and workplans; (iv) to maintain the organisational philosophy, there will be increased need for the leader to discuss and monitor individuals' work.

Possible strategies include: (i) scheduled reviews of staff experiences and programme progress; (ii) regular planning of SIAAP and individual work programmes; (iii) learning to say 'no' to some requests; (iv) maintaining a focus on quality (by setting quality goals and regularly monitoring and discussing quality achievements); (v) the leader may need to maintain a focus on setting priorities, planning, and monitoring quality whilst beginning to delegate implementation and supervision.

Discussion Question 3:

What impact did donor funding have on SIAAP? What steps could SIAAP take to minimise the disadvantages of accepting external funding? What strategies might SIAAP use to further develop the support it gets from local sources?

(a) Impact on SIAAP

- All donor funding is accompanied by donor agency regulations. The WHO partnership programme required that SIAAP find an organisational partner.
- Donor agencies have their own approval procedures before funds are allocated. In this case, SIAAP suffered because the anticipated funds from the Partnership Programme did not materialise. Shyamla had to find other funds, from family and friends, to keep the workshop programme on track.
- Even following approval, donor funding may take a long time to arrive. SIAAP had to wait a considerable time before the Ford Foundation money was available to them in Madras.
- Donors require regular and systematic accounting of expenditures. SIAAP is having to look for help in maintaining their financial records and producing their financial reports.
- Donors usually require periodic progress reports on the project being supported. SIAAP is also having to consider hiring secretarial help.

(b) Minimising the Disadvantages of External Funding:

- SIAAP could establish criteria tor those areas that could be financed by donors and those which should be financed by community. e.g. SIAAP could decide that investment costs were provided by donors, while they will attempt to fund recurrent costs by contributions from the community.
- Other steps that SIAAP might decitle to take include: setting ceilings for the maximum amount of external funding that it will accept; setting time limits for the period for external funding;

(iii) careful selection of the donors, based on previous experience, donor conditions, etc; restricting the number of donors at any one time; (iv) diversifying the donors, so that SIAAP is not reliant upon a single source of external funding.

(c) Strategies for Local Fund-raising:

Strategies that SIAAP could use include: using personal contacts (both individuals and organisations) to seek support; identifying whether fees could be charged for SIAAP services; seeking for ways in which the communities served can make in-kind contributions; conducting regular or special collection campaigns; investigating the possibility of obtaining Government grants; conducting research on private sector organisations to identify their interests (and their skills), and develop targetted proposals for their support; targetting citizens overseas for contributions.

Discussion Question 4:

What recommendations would you make to Shyamla and the team on how they might continue to develop their programmes in the future?

Some possibilities include:

(i) clarification of SIAAP's mission and priorities. (Perhaps reestablishing NGO support as priority. Much more could be done if as many NGOs as possible were capable of contributing to the HIV/AIDS problem, so it might be more effective in the long run for SIAAP to help others than to try and do things themselves.); (ii) recruiting individuals with specific skills to SIAAP so that individuals could specialise in helping NGOs in certain interventions; (iii) careful monitoring of the effectiveness of the NGO support programme; (iv) seeking to develop "apex" NGOs in different locations so that these could also begin to act as resources (technical/materials) to other NGOs; (v) prioritisation of activities within the limits of SIAAP's capacity (learning to say "no" to some requests for assistance); (vi) seeking to support SIAAP leadership by looking for strong deputies to ensure smooth succession.

8

Marketing NGO/Business Sector Partnerships

JAMES P. REINNOLDT

Regional Managing Director for Thailand Indochina and West Asia at Northwest Airlines, Inc.

THE ROLE OF MARKETING

Efficient application of marketing principles provides the firm with a competitive advantage. In other words, it is able to use its resources more effectively than other firms, thereby becoming more profitable. Marketing helps the firm in the following ways:

1. By producing an integrated view of the entire market, which allows for the development of an effective long-term strategy. *What can the firm achieve?*
2. By defining medium-term investment oriteria to invest in new products or services. *Where are the greatest opportunities?*
3. By positioning both new and old products or services to achieve the best result consistent with the long-term strategy. *How can the firm take advantage of those opportunities?*

In summary, the adherence to a business philosophy which always put the needs and wants of the customer first wvill help bring about a dynamic and pro-active stance that allows a firm to formulate and execute effective and profitable business strategies.

MARKET SEGMENTATION

The original definition of marketing here included "...the fulfilling of consumers' needs and wants". It was also noted that market oriented firms focus the development and delivery of their products and services on the basis-above all-of their needs.

As the marketer cannot possibly hope to satisfy *all* needs of *all* the customers, he must instead try to determine to which group he can sell his product most profitably. This need-based grouping is called market segmentation.

"A market segment is a group of customers who have sufficient in common to form a suitable basis for a product/price/distribution/ promotion combination. This market segment becomes a target group."

The driving reason behind market segmentation is so that marketers may most effectively allocate resources to achieve their objectives. It provides marketing "economies of scale". It is important to strike a balance here, however. A firm cannot afford to segment the total market too finely or he will lose the essential cost effectiveness. For example, should he group and pursue a group of 300 students who travel each year? On the other hand, he cannot afford to define the market too broadly. This "undersegmentation" will result in a poor estimation and assessment of a group's needs- and fail to make the right marketing pitch.

WHAT IS THE MARKETING MIX?

Marketing has been defined as activities involved with the satisfaction of wants and needs. These activities combine to make the marketing process. More commonly they are known as the marketing mix or the "four Ps":

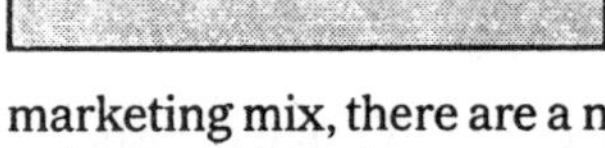

The combination of these four activities constitute the *marketing mix.* They are interdependent activities; that is, they are most effectively applied in a concerted, combined effort or strategy.

For each component of the marketing mix, there are a number of decisions to be made, or factors to be considered:

PRODUCT DECISIONS:

- What should be supplied?
- What brands should be used?
- How should it be styled or designed?
- In what quantity should it be produced?
- In what way can it be used?

WHAT IS MARKETING

Marketing can be defined in a number of ways. Most commonly it is considered as the fulfilling of consumer needs at a profit to the organization. More specifically it demands an understanding of the market factors such as how the law, government, competition, or structure of the market will affect what the firm is trying to achieve, what is preferred by potential customers, and the implications of producing and selling the item that is involved.

"Marketing is human activity directed at satisfying needs and wants through exchange processes". (Philip Kotler)

Traditionally, firms were involved with management, administration and production, the latter of which became most important following the industrial revolution which saw the introduction of new manufacturing processes that led to the inexpensive and mass production of various products. At that time, manufacturing was the key, and the marketplace craved the supply of anything new; it was a 'seller's market" where the producer was king.

PRODUCTION-THINKING ASKS "WHAT SHALL WE MAKE?"

Once the markets became saturated with goods that exceeded consumer demand, manufacturing firms began searching for ways to distinguish their products from those of the competition. In doing so, they asked the consumer what he needed. Thus, the marketing revolution was born.

MARKETING-THINKING ASKS "WHAT DOES THE CONSUMER WANT?"

The understanding of consumer wants and needs is actually a multi-faceted process. It involves the understanding of:

- Who is the consumer?
- Where is the customer?
- What is important to him/her?

MARKETING BEGINS AND ENDS WITH THE CUSTOMER." MATCHING THE NEEDS WITH THE PRODUCT

NEED:	Reduce employer's staff-related costs.
PRODUCT:	AIDS Awareness Prograrn for employees.
TARGET AUDIENCE:	Finance and Human Resource Managers

NEED:	Enhance Employee Morale
PRODUCT:	Assistance with development of AIDS personnel policies. Employee education and awareness.

TARGET AUDIENCE:	Human Resource Managers
NEED:	Enhanced corporate image. Public relations.
PRODUCT:	Opportunity for firm to join coalition against AIDS. Involvement in social and community issues.
TARGET AUDIENCE:	Marketing and Public Relations Managers.
NEED:	Social Responsibility.
PRODUCT:	Opportunity to make donation to worthy cause.
TARGET AUDIENCE:	General Managers

WHAT ARE THE NEEDS OF THE PRIVATE SECTOR?

1. Financial
- Employee Turnover
- Insurance Premiums

2. Internal
- Employee Morale
- Employee Educations and Development

3. Promotional
- Public Relations
- Corporate Image
- Advertising

4. Social
- Social Responsibility

The Marketing Process

1. Conduct Research	Direct-Mall Survey to Business Associations Reveals that 67% of Respondents have little or no knowledge of AIDS, and a lack of training programs.
2. Set Objectives	Assist 150 firms in Thailand with the creation of an AIDS awareness program in 1992.
3. Identify Targets	H.R. Managers in 465 American, 102 Canadian and 145 British firms in Bangkok.

4. Determine Strategy	Create an AIDS awareness day Campaign for Target firms.
5. Define Tactics	- Speak to chamber luncheon. - Invite target audience to seminar. - Follow-up with phone calls and letters. - Make Appointments and office visits. - Launch AIDS awareness day.
6. Program Review	Review success of program. Lessons learned.

UNDERSTANDING THE NEEDS OF YOUR MARKET (RESEARCH)

"Consumer-oriented marketing begins with a keen understanding of the customer's needs and wants in order that the product can be tailored to satisfy those wants."

SOURCES OF INFORMATION:

Chamber of Commerce Guides:
- Size of Firm.
- Names/addresses of managers.
- Types of business.

Annual Reports:
- Corporate Mission Statement.
- Corporate Philosophy.

Public Relations Departments:
- History of gift-giving.
- Recent community involvement.

Surveys:
- Size of firms.
- Philosophy.
- Interest in various products.
- Extent of on-going AIDS programs.

Learning Points

1. Marketing is comprised of those activities involved with the satisfaction of needs and wants. It is a process; a means to an end.
2. While the business sector may have its own culture and set of rules, its basic needs are the same as the rest of society. People are at the core.
3. The business sector needs the help of NGOs in order to minimize the impact of HIV and AIDS on its customers and employees.

4. In order to achieve successful NGO/business partnerships, NGOs and the business sector must understand the needs of the other party, respect their differences and compensate for their weaknesses.
5. NGO/business partnerships must be approached by means of a goal-oriented strategic process which includes establishing goals, conducting research, setting specific objectives, identifying targets, determining strategy, defining tactics and reviewing the process.
6. The needs of the business sector include financial (e.g., employee turnover), internal (e.g., employee morale), promotional (e.g., public relations) and social (e.g., social responsibility) needs.
7. NGOs can obtain backgraound information on business from the Chamber of Commerce Guides, Annual Reports, public relations departments and business surveys.
8. The power and effectiveness of NGO/business partnerships are much greater than the sum of each working alone.

9

HIV in the Workplace

INTRODUCTION

Adults between the ages of 15 - 35 are the group most affected by HIV and AIDS. It is estimated that approximately 90 per cent of the persons suffering from AIDS/ARC (AIDS related complex) or infected with HIV are in the labour force. Thus it is clear that HIV and AIDS can have a devastating effect on the economy, directly through the loss of skilled and unskilled labour, and indirectly through increased costs of medical care.

As AIDS enters the workplace, government agencies, companies and labour unions are all struggling to develop strategies to respond to the issues being faced, including: lost productivity; employee turnover; hiring policies; increased medical costs; employee benefits; HIV testing; customer relations; confidentiality of medical information; confidentiality and discrimination against HIV-infected employees.

POLICY ISSUES

In 1988 the WHO, in collaboration with the International Labour Organization, participated in a consultation on AIDS and the Workplace. The participants included representatives from government, unions, business, public health, and the medical and legal professions of 18 countries. The following fundamental principles emerged from the consultation:

1. Workers with HIV-related illnesses, including AIDS, should be treated in the same way as any other worker with any other illness.
2. People living with HIV and AIDS should be allowed to continue working in a supportive workplace setting if they so desire.
3. Comprehensive health promotion and appropriate workplace policies help provide an opportunity to create an atmosphere conducive to caring for and promoting the health of all workers and are essential for effective HIV prevention programs.
4. In the vast majority of workplace settings, work does not involve any risk of the HIV infection being transmitted between co-workers or between workers and clients.
5. Pre-employment HIV-antibody screening to assess a person's fitness to work is unnecessary and should not be required.

The initial reaction of employers in many countries to the possibility of HIV infection in their companies has been to screen potential employees for HIV-infection. However, preemployment HIV screening is both costly and ineffective.

HIV infection is not a reason for terminating employment. Persons with HIV-related illnesses can and should be allowed to continue as productive members of the workforce as long as they are medically fit. Furthermore, screening for HIV is not a preventive measure.

WORK PLACE EDUCATION

When an employee is suspected or diagnosed as having HIV or AIDS, a wave of fear, panic and confusion often ensue in the workplace.

The disruption can be minimized by providing HIV education and support services to all employees and by establishing HIV related personnel policies in advance.

The advantages of a workplace AIDS education program include: the promotion of higher worker productivity; maintaining the health and welfare of employees; establishing clarity concerning legal issues; developing a consistent company policy; and promoting a positive company image. Successful models of workplace AIDS programs already exist in the Asia and Pacific region.

A workplace AIDS program must be supported by management at all levels in order to succeed. Management support lends credibility to the program and provides a strong incentive for others to follow. Managers themselves must know enough about HIV/AIDS to give informed responses to the concerns of their subordinates. They must also be fully aware of the company policy pertaining to HIV and AIDS.

The purpose of educating the workforce about HIV/AIDS is to reduce fear, diffuse prejudice, avoid panic and disruption, disseminate factual information, and to maintain stability and productivity.

The following issues must be addressed in order to meet these objectives: the medical realities of AIDS; the fact that employees are not at risk of contracting HIV infection during routine workplace activities; company policy concerning AIDS; acknowledgement of concerns and fears; management's willingness to communicate with them and hear their concerns; and that other companies are dealing with AIDS in the workplace.

Fear can be expected as an initial response to AIDS or any new disease. When an employee expresses fear about AIDS, it is important to acknowledge and validate that fear. If fear and concern about AIDS are dismissed, ignored or put down, they will increase and ultimately become larger problems.

Employees will want to know the corporate policy on AIDS. Clear communication of company policy concerning AIDS is a statement to employees as to where the company stands on the AIDS issues. It is a strong inducement for employees to work through their own issues concerning AIDS.

Barriers to workplace-based . AIDS programs which must be overcome include: employers' difficulty in dealing with sensitive issues such as sexuality, drugs and death; apathy about AIDS; fear, ignorance and denial of the epidemic; lack of financial resources; and a lack of knowledge of what to do.

Workplace programs are of critical importance in minimizing the social and economic costs of the HIV epidemic. The workplace provides a unique challenge and opportunity to provide support for HIV-infected individuals, reduce discrimination and fear of HIV and AIDS and to prevent the further spread of the virus.

Principles for Responding to AIDS in the Workplace

1. People with HIV infection or AIDS are entitled to the same rights and opportunities as people with other serious or life-threatening illness.
2. Employment policies should be based on the scientific and epidemiological evidence that people with AIDS or HIV infection do not pose a risk of transmitting the virus to co-workers or clients through ordinary workplace contact.
3. The highest levels of management and employee organisation leaders should endorse non-discriminatory

employment policies and workplace AIDS education and support programs.

4. Employers and employee organisations should communicate their support of these policies to workers in simple, clear and unambiguous terms.
5. Employers should provide employees with sensitive, accurate, and up-to-date education about risk reduction in their personal lives.
6. Employers have a duty to protect the confidentiality of employees' medical information.
7. To prevent work disruption and rejection by co-workers of an employee with HIV-infection or AIDS, employers and employee organisations should undertake education for all employees before such an incident occurs and as needed thereafter.
8. Employers should not require HIV screenng as part of general pre-employment or workplace physical examinations.
9. In those special occupational settings where there may be a potential risk of exposure to HIV (for example, in health care, where workers may be exposed to blood or blood products), employers should provide specific on-going eduction and training, as well as the necessary equipment, to reinforce appropriate infection control procedures and ensure that they are implemented.

10

HIV: The Legal Issues

INTRODUCTION

There is currently some resistance within the legal profession to view HIV and AIDS as a legitimate human rights issue. There have been attempts to block research on AIDS-related legal issues and there is a tendency among legislators to see AIDS as "causing trouble" in the formulation and implementation of national development plans.

However, a multitude of human rights violations have been documented in relationship to people with HIV and AIDS. Frequent violations which have been documented globally include:

- Mandatory testing of employees for HIV;
- Dismissal of employees suspected of being, or diagnosed as, HIV positive;
- Breaches of confidentiality through the disclosure of employees' HIV status;
- Discrimination, against individuals who are perceived to be at high risk for HIV infection, such as migrant or foreign worlcers.

While the law cannot solve all the problems related to the epidemic, it can help create a supportive environment for people living with HIV and AIDS. The law can provide a clear framework to direct the public and private sectors to be more responsible and more responsive to the needs of those affected by the epidemic.

Many nations have considered the adoption of a pecific AIDS Law. The necessity and apropriateness of such a law has been the focus of much discussion and debate. In the absence of a cure, or vaccine, the only means of prevention open to us is through individual behavior change. Howeva, experience has consistently demonstrated that legislation alone is insufficient to change behaviour.

Another argument for a specific AIDS law is to ensure the rights of individuals living with HIV and AIDS. However, it may be that an AIDS specific law is not necessary, but that HIV and AIDS should be incorporated within or covered by other legislation.

LABOUR LAW

Labour law generally applies only to the formal sector and does not cover the informal sectors such as seasonal or migratory labour and rural employment. Therefore, many people remain unprotected. It is imperative that we find ways to reach these people.

Workplace issues which can be addressed by pre-existing or newly-created legislation include: screening of employees for HIV infection; confidentiality; discriminatory, hiring and dismissal of infected individuals; and medical benefits to infected individuals.

For example, with regard to the issue of medical benefits for HIV infected employees, guidance can be sought from pre-existing legislation such as Civil Law, Social Security Acts and Workmen's Compensation Schemes.

THE BUSINESS SECTOR AND LAW

Laws can be used to encourage the business sector to become actively involved in HIV education and support activities. For example, legislation can be enacted which provides a tax exemption to businesses engaged in HIV and AIDS-related activities; social security legislation can be expanded to provide benefits to businesses which employ HIV-infected individuals and existing human rights legislation can be expanded to protect the rights of people living with HIV and AIDS.

CONCLUSION

In order to respond effectively to the challenges posed by HIV and AIDS, all sectors and strata of society will need to be mobilized. While we should not depend on law to solve the problems related to HIV and AIDS, the law can be used as a complementary tool to minimize the social and economic impact of the epidemic.

Although in certain situations and countries, new AIDS-specific laws may need to be created or existing laws extended to specifically address HIV and AIDS, these laws must be developed cautiously. Otherwise, the laws may have unintended consequences.

For example, one draft AIDS Law developed in Thailand in 1991 provided additional social security for people living with HIV, but also gave the authorities the right to detain HIV infected persons.

Country specific analysis will need to be conducted to assess the utility and cost effectiveness of developing AIDS-specific legislation. It is possible that the resources necessary to develop and implement such a law would be better used in other ways, e.g., promotion of AIDS education in work places.

The primary use of law in AIDS should be to guarantee the rights of people living with HIV and AIDS.

LEARNING POINTS

General Legal Issues

1. Laws alone are not enough to bring about the individual attitude and behaviour change required to prevent the further spread of HIV.
2. The law can be used as a tool to promote and create a supportive social and political environment for people living with HIV and AIDS, e.g., legislation prohibiting the discrimination against people living with HIV and AIDS in the workplace.
3. In considering the development and implementation of new legislation pertaining to HIV and AIDS, careful consideration should be given to the actual impact of the law on the human rights of people living with HIV and AIDS.
4. In using the legal system to advocate for the rights of people living with HIV and AIDS, one must understand that the judiciary is influenced by the general social, political and economic environment in which it functions.

Legal Issues for NGO/Business Partnerships

1. Legislation can be used to encurage businesses to create a supportive environment for people living with HIV and AIDS, e.g., tax incentives for businesses which employ people living with HIV. However, legislation will not change the attitudes and behaviour of individuals.
2. NGOs and businesses should be knowledgeable about the implications of pre-existing public health, labour and other laws for HIV and AIDS related workplace issues. For example, the right of HIV-infected people and those with AIDS to social security, social and medical assistance, or social welfare services may be covered under existing legislation.

3. NGOs should be knowledgeable about the legal framework for workplace issues, such as, screening, confidentiality and discrimination when working with a business to develop HIV and AIDS-related personnel policies.

11

HIV: Social Security and Insurance Schemes

PROF. NIKOM CHANDRAVITHUN
Thamsart University, Bangkok, Thailand

The idea of social security was originaily conceived over 100 years ago in Germany. As countries move from family agricultural systems to a wage system, traditional family-based forms of social support tend to become eroded. The loss of income from employment due to disability, sickness, etc. will therefore result in greater hardship. Social security is intended as a safety net to offset this loss of income. In addition, social security is a means of spreading the increasing cost of medical care between rich and poor, between healthy and unhealthy, and between people who live long lives and those who die prematurely.

The benefits of social security are that workers receive guaranteed security, employers get a contented and healthier work force, and society gets social stability. It is not a step towards socialism, but a way to make capitalism more acceptable.

In terms of finance, social security is a large operation. Although figures are not available for the developing countries, the experience in the developed world with social security spending indicates that a large and growing proportion of the GDP is allocated to social security spending. For example, as a percentage of GDP, Australia spends 9%, Austria 24%, Canada 16%, Japan 11%, and the UK 19% on social security. This is largely because of high health expenditure, e.g., Australia 7%, UK 6%, and the USA 11% of GDP.

Even before the advent of HIV, health expenditure had already reached high levels in industrialized countries.

In Thailand we have been trying to work out what impact HIV will have on the level of social security payments. So far we have not reached any definite conclusions. At the moment workers in the formal sector are entitled to 12 months' social security on half pay, but it seems that after that period the government would have to come in and provide assistance.

The most cost-effective solution is prevention of HIV/AIDS. Business leaders have a responsibility to educate their employees about AIDS prevention. In terms of medical care, the pharmaceutical industry should be prepared to contribute as well.

I want to congratulate UNDP for their initiative on this issue, and I hope this meeting will be only the beginning of this very important exercise.

LEARNING POINTS

Benefits of Social Security

1. Benefits to workers include: a sense of security and a gurantee that minimal survival needs will be met.
2. Benefits to employers include: a more contented and healthier workforce.
3. The primary benefit to society in providing social security and insurance schemes is overall social stability.

Impact of HIV and AIDS on Social Security and Insurance Schemes

1. HIV and AIDS will have a cost impact on the provision of social security and insurance schemes in any country which experiences a high incidence of HIV and AIDS.
2. The increased cost of providing social security and insurance benefits will require the support of both the public and private sectors.
3. Creative strategies to care for people affected by HIV-related illness will need to be adopted in order to cope with prohibitive costs associated with hospital based care.
4. Prevention of HIV infection through education and behaviour change is the most cost-effective means of minimizing the cost to society of the HIV epidemic.

12

Private Sector Collaboration on AIDS Prevention

JOHN BAKER
Project Director

INTRODUCTION

The Population and Community Development Association (PDA) established a comprehensive HIV/AIDS prevention programme in 1989 under the premise that AIDS prevention in Thailand required active participation from all sectors of society, especially the private business sector. Recognizing that the private sector had much to offer AIDS prevention, PDA solicited the involvement of a variety of companies to perform specific roles. PDA's AIDS prevention program also relied upon important cooperation with other non-conventional sectors and organizations, such as the Royal Thai Army and the Ministry of Interior.

PDA's collaboration with companies includes a diverse range of activities which can be categorized into four main groups:

(1) Company service to PDA
(2) Company service to community
(3) PDA service to company
(4) Collaborative effort serving PDA, company and community.

Companies became involved for a variety of reasons and the respective collaborative efforts came about by different means. While it is difficult to generalize from PDA's experience for the benefit of other NGOs, some basic principles for successful NGO-company partnerships can be identified. NGOs must recognize their own needs in order to identify a suitable corporate partner; NGOs must recognize the needs of their prospective corporate partner to manage a successful relationship; and NGOs must conduct the relationship in a professional manner to ensure full cooperation from the corporate partner.

PDA AND AIDS IN THAILAND

The Population and Community Development Association (PDA) was established in 1974 by Mechai Viravaidya to provide family planning services throughout Thailand. Using a system of community volunteer distributors, PDA served 16,000 (one third of all) villages in Thailand by 1978. Recognizing that acceptance of family planning was a function of other factors such as health and income, PDA integrated a range of other services along with family planning. Health education, parasite control, latrine and drinking water storage tank construction, agricultural credit and extension, water resources development, community forestry, and community institution-building now form the bulk of PDA's programs along with family planning.

PDA's AIDS prevention program has evolved with the changing epidemic in Thailand since 1987. Today, about 600,000 Thais are HIVpositive and this number increases by about 1,000-1,300 infections per day mostly through heterosexual intercourse. Such widespread HIV infection has grown at a rapid pace since 1988.

PDA entered into AIDS prevention in 1987 by anticipating HIV spread among commercial sex workers in Bangkok and Pattaya. Expanding upon a family planning and STD prevention education programme to commercial sex establishments (mostly massage parlors) in Bangkok and up-country, PDA implemented an operations research project. The objective of the project was to determine the effectiveness of peer educators in certain commercial sex enterprises (gay bars, go-go bars and massage parlors) to change the knowledge, attitudes and behavior with regard to HIV infection of other commercial sex workers in those establishments.

By late 1988, HIV prevalence among such commercial sex workers remained minimal but the HIV infection growth rates arnong IVDUs in Banglcok exploded from 1% in early 1988 to 32-43% in September 1988. This information confirmed the importance of PDA's comprehensive AIDS prevention programme. Already, PDA maintained that AIDS was not a health problem but a-societal problem, and thus required a societal response including all sectors of society. PDA's first major effort was the Private Sector Initiative in AIDS Prevention in 1989, since then private sector collaborations have been critical to AIDS prevention activities in Thailand.

With the need to rapidly educate Thai society about HIV/AIDS at a time when the government was reluctant to allow high visibility of such information in the mass media, PDA approached Ogilvy & Mather advertising agency to produce some television and radio spots quickly, professionally and inexpensively. O&M obliged and produced four TV spots and eight radio spots at cost. PDA then prevailed upon the Supreme Commander of the Armed Forces to air these spots on the two TV networks and 400 radio stations controlled by the military. One of the radio spots earned O&M an award for best public service advertisement. The military also adopted a PDA recommendation to care for any military personnel or immediate family members infected with HIV.

To begin educating groups of people about HIV/AIDS, PDA needed high quality audio-visual materials. With the assistance of Kodak, PDA produced an 80-slide slide show together with a synchronized audio tape and a manual to be distributed throughout the country. As all local governrnents from the provincial down to the village level are administered through the Ministry of Interior, PDA collaborated with them to train all provincial governors and district officers on HIV/AIDS. In addition, PDA trained all Director Generals in the Ministry of the Interior which includes the Police Deparanent, the Labor Department, and other important departments.

To reach a wider audience with printed AIDS education materials, PDA invited the cooperation of a number of companies with large customer bases and highly visible profiles. American International Assurance printed AIDS information-for distribution to their millions of life insurance policy-holders. PDA also distributed these materials to other audiences. Krating Daeng, manufacturer of a widely popular and available electrolyte beverage, printed AIDS information which was distributed along with their product. Avon, the direct sales cosmetic company, printed AIDS information for distribution through their direct sales force and promoted AIDS awareness through several sales promotion events. All of these materials were also available to PDA for distribution to the general public.

Upon learning of the magnitude of the AIDS situation in Thailand from PDA's Chairman, Mechai Viravaidya, on a TV talk show, an executive vice-president of Thai Farmers Bank (TFB) asked him to discuss the realities of AIDS in Thailand with the bank's executive committee. The bank responded to the business reasons why Thailand's second largest bank should actively help to prevent the spread of AIDS and agreed to collaborate with PDA on a proposed $200,000 program including the following components:

(1) PDA provides AIDS education to TFB staff;

(2) TFB supports PDA's economic impact of AIDS on Thailand analysis;
(3) PDA briefs TFB's top 200 corporate clients on the realities of AIDS in Thailand;
(4) TFB supports economic assistance to five villages in Northern Thailand where women are known to enter prostitution;
(5) TFB supports PDA HIV/AIDS counselling services.

PDA has engaged with many other companies in AIDS prevention and corporate collaboration is important to PDA's AIDS prevention programme. PDA also educates corporate staff on AIDS in the workplace programmes. Many companies have donated funds for AIDS education activities. Minnesota Mining and Manufacturing (3M) provided generous supplies of video and audio tapes for the replication of AIDS education materials.

TYPES OF PRIVATE SECTOR COLLABORATIONS:

PDA's collaborations with companies on AIDS prevention include a diverse range of activities and can be categorized into four main groups.

(a) Company service to PDA

In the initial stages of the rapid spread of HIV izn Thailand, PDA needed the resources and skills of the private sector to disseminate effective AIDS education messages. PDA relied upon the services of the Ogilvy & Mather advertising agency and the resources of Kodak in providing slide sets and 3M in providing video and audio tapes. In these cases, PDA provided public relations benefits to these companies but the companies' conscience and goodwill in these instances were noteworthy.

Certainly, the beneficiaries of such generosity were the general public where PDA played the role of facilitator.

(b) Company service to community

Where companies donated AIDS information materials printed with their logos and corporate identities (as in the cases of AIA, Krating Daeng and Avon mentioned above), the beneficiaries were also the general public. The companies also intended informing their customer base about AIDS.

(c) PDA service to company

PDA educates corporate staff and conducts in-depth training for company representatives on AIDS. Companies usually offer an unsolicited donation to PDA in appreciation for the service. Of course, the motivation in this situation is to protect their staff by arranging the necessary educational services.

(d) Collaborative effort serving PDA company and community

Where PDA presented a large corporate entity with a comprehensive AIDS prevention programme proposal, Thai Farmers Bank genuinely engaged in an exchange package of service, skills and resources for the benefit of their company, PDA's programmes, and the community.

NGO-BUSINESS COLLABORATION STRATEGIES

There are certain principles and strategies which may help NGOs conduct successful relationships with private businesses in AIDS prevention.

(1) Recognize your (NGO) needs.

NGOs must recognize their own needs in order to identify a suitable corporate partner. In order to implement the NGO's plan, what is required from the private sector: skills, resources (material, human, financial), connections, a wider audience (customers), etc.?

(2) Recognize company needs and interests.

NGOs must recognize the needs and interests of their prospective corporate partner to manage a successful relationship. What does the company want in exchange for its collaboration: public relations, introductions, goodwill with the government or general public, etc.?

(3) Be professional

NGOs must conduct the relationship in a most professional manner to ensure full cooperation from the corporate partner.

(4) Use personal contacts

Personal contacts are an effective means of establishing a successful relationship with a company. Invite corporate executives onto the NGO's Board, attend Chamber of Commerce meetings, provide a service which the corporate sector needs, etc.

LEARNING POINTS

1. Partnerships are based on a common understanding of each partners interest and expectation of benefits. In the case of HIV the mutual interest is in responding to the epidemic. Although the response of each partner might arise from different motivations, the objective of each

partner would be to prevent the further spread of HIV and to minimize the effects of existing infections.

2. The prerequisite for establishing any partnership is mutual respect. In addition to a common language and understanding of the goals of the partnership, the organizations must trust each other's competence and commnitment to the partnership. For NGOs this means acting in a professional manner with clear objectives, accountability and delivery of promised goals. For businesses this means being clear about motives and the extent and type of support which they can offer the NGO.

3. Partnerships should be built on existing commitment and interest. It is not essential for the business to be motivated by humanitarian goals. Similarly, NGOs do not have to relinquish their social goals to work with the business sector. As long as the different motivations of the partners are acknowledge and respected, both parties can work together toward a common goal.

4. Develop and make use of personal relationships. Both private sector business and NGO networking depends on effective personal relationships. Personal relationships should be consciously cultivated in partnerships, friendships are the most productive partnerships, they should be preserved even when there is no immediate benefit. Once established network can be productive in the long term in ways which were not apparent at the outset.

5. NGOs can provide guidance to businesses in developing work-based AIDS education and policies to reduce the spread of the virus and minimize the impact of the epidemic on the business.

6. It is important for NGOs to recognize the constraints of the business in developing and implementing approapriate responses to HIV and AIDS in the workplace. Businesses will often require some time to fully implement HIV prevention and support programmes. The need for time should not necessarily be perceived as lack of commitment of failure.

13

Succesful Partnerships: Action for AIDS -Saatchi and Saatchi Advertising Singapore

ROY CHAN
Member, Action for AIDS
Singapore

BILL TIMMERMAN
Saatchi and Saatchi Advertising
Singapore

The relationship between Action for AIDS Singapore (AfA) and Saatchi & Saatchi began in November of 1990 when a member of AfA approached Saatchi & Saatchi to request assistance in producing an advertisement for the 1990 World AIDS Day. The theme of World AIDS Day that year was "Women and AIDS".

Saatchi & Saatchi not only agreed to donate its services to produce the World AIDS Day advertisement, but also created two additional advertisements in magazines. This first effort broke new ground, being the first advertisement in Singapore to feature condoms.

Since then Saatchi & Saatchi has created two more campaigns for AfA, as well as other materials such as a gay men's booklet and packaging for condom distribution. Saatchi & Saatchi also redesigned AfA's logo and stationery.

One of Saatchi & Saatchi's motivations in donating its services to AfA was the belief that advertising agencies have a particularly important role to play in the fight against AIDS. This is because of the high degree of direct control individuals can exercise over the amount of risk to which they are willing to subject themselves. Effective advertising which motivates changes in behaviour is one of few weapons against AIDS available at this time.

As an NGO, AfA cannot begin to match the financial and human resources of government organizations such as the Singapore Ministry of Health. But, as an NGO, it has fewer constraints on what it can say and do. One of the primary objectives of the AfA/Saatchi & Saatchi partnership is, therefore, to complement the efforts of the Ministry of Health, including breaking new ground in AIDS awareness advertising.

The relationship has been mutually beneficial. For AfA, the advertising has helped raise and shape public opinion, raise credibility of AfA, maximize AfA's resources, and "market" the message. For Saatchi & Saatchi, it has helped boost employee morale, and is an opportunity to do award winning advertising as well as to use the agency's skills for a truly worthwhile cause. The agency believes that donating its services to AfA and other such causes also has business benefits in terms of helping to attract like minded talent and clients.

LEARNING POINTS

Facilitating Factors for Successful Partnerships

1. Professionalism. The ability of NGOs to provide services in a timely and "professional" manner.
2. Presentation. The ability of NGOs to present their proposal and organization to the business. In particular, their ability to illustrate the benefit of collaboration (financial or non financial) to the business.
3. Credibility. The NGO should present a clear description of their skills and experience record to the business.
4. Mutual benefits. Partnerships should be mutually beneficial for the NGO and the business.
5. Focus. The NGO should have a concrete proposal including the substance and scope of the collaboration it seeks with the business.
6. Mutual respect. Understanding and acceptance of each others "corporate culture" is necessary for good working relationships.
7. Social mandate of business. Pre-existing concern and willingness of business to be involved in HIV and AIDS activities.
8. Social context. The existence of a positive social, political and legal environment in regard to individuals living with HIV and AIDS.

14

Characteristics of Partnerships: The NGO Perspective

TERESITA MARIE P. BAGASAO
Core Member
International Council of AIDS Service Organisations in Asia and the Pacific

BACKGROUND

The role of non-government organizations (NGOs) in the fight against AIDS has been recognized worldwide. Yet many NGOs may lack the resources needed to undertake prevention and care programmes that could have lasting impact and sustainability.

Traditionally, NGOs have relied on support from government, development assistance groups and other donor agencies. With the magnitude of the AIDS epidemic, there is a need to go beyond traditional partnerships and venture into new ones.

The private business sector has been known to provide support to NGOs. In AIDS, this has happened in countries where the epidemic is visible and widespread. What has happened to other countries where AIDS is not as visible or known? This short study tries to seek some answers based on the NGO perspective.

In particular, the study hopes to provide information on perception, attitudes and actual experiences of NGOs with regards to developing partnerships with the business sector for AIDS education, prevention and care.

The study was jointly conducted by Action for AIDS, Singapore and Kabalikat ng Pamilyang Pilipino for presentation at this consultation. It is by no means representative of the entire NGO community but provides some idea based on a sub-sample drawn from NGOs in the Asia and Pacific region working on AIDS. Fourteen (14) NGOs from Hong Kong, Indonesia, Malaysia, Philippines, Singapore and Thailand agreed to answer the two page questionnaire (Appendix A) which included questions about the NGOs and their AIDS activities, motivation, attitude, and experience in working with private business.

DESCRIPTION OF NGOs

The 14 NGOs surveyed are working on AIDS education and almost all provide some counselling services Cable 1). The audience/ clients served by these NGOs vary, but the majority world with women, gay/bisexual men and sex workers (Table 2).

NGOs PERCEPTION OF WORKING WITH THE BUSINESS SECTOR

All of the NGOs surveyed stated that funding was the primary motivation for working with the business sector. Equipment and other material resources were named as the second (Table 3). The NGOs saw themselves as providing business information and education either to the business staff or clients and providing some form of product endorsement (Table 4).

NGO EXPERIENCE WITH BUSINESS

Eight of the NGOs surveyed, have collaborated with business. Activities include fund raising for NGO concerns; providing public education on issues undertaken by NGOs; providing some kind of publicity for both NGO and business (Table 5). To initiate contact with business, these NGOs had to develop a programme that could be sold to the business. This may be linked to their perception of business primarily as a source of funding support. However, there were some NGOs who assisted businesses to analyze their policy on AIDS and further explored the kind of AIDS programmes these businesses were willing to support (Table 6).

Factors which reportedly facilitated NGO/business partnerships include: the track record of the NGO and their "professionalism"; their credibility; the recognition of mutual benefits for both parties and the continuous interpersonal relationship brought about by good follow-up by NGOs with their business partners (Table 7).

However, these NGO/business partnerships were not without their difficulties. Common problems encountered by NGOs in initiating and maintaining successful collaborations were business managements' receptivity to AIDS as an issue, which may or may not be related to what the NGOs perceive as business ignorance and denial of the relevance of AIDS (Table 8).

CONCLUSION

From this brief survey, we can conclude that NGOs working on AIDS have not looked at business as a target or client but continue to look at them as a source of support. The other point that may need further discussion is that the onus of initiation on collaboration on AIDS seems to be on the NGO. Considering this, how then does an NGO actually prepare itself to work with business? What kinds of knowledge and skills will be necessary for NGOs to acquire or strengthen to make partnerships with business work? The concrete examples by the panelists from India, Philippines and Thailand may help us define these issues.

SURVEY RESULTS

Presentation by: Teresita Bagasao, Kabalikat, Philippines Roy Chan, Action for AIDS, Singapore

TABLE 1: TYPE OF NGO ACTIVITIES

Education	14
Counselling	12
HIV Testing	4
Welfare/Care	5
Networking	1
Prof/Tech Assistance	2

TABLE 2: TARGET GROUPS

Sex Workers	7
Women	9
Gay/Bisexual Men	8
Intravenous Drug Users	3
Youth	5
Health Care Workers	2
Others	5

TABLE 3: NGOS' PERCEPTION OF BUSINESS ASSISTANCE

Funding	14
Equipment	9
Time	1
Services	1

{Cont.}...

Marketing of NGO	3
Expertise	4
Access to Employees	1
Public relations	1
Networking	2
IEC to Public	3

TABLE 4: NGOS' PERCEPTION OF THEIR ASSISTANCE TO BUSINESS

IEC to Staff	9
IEC to Clients	5
Product Endorsement	8
Product Consumption	1
Product Distribution	1
Public Relations	3
Market Research	3
HIV Guidelines	1

TABLE 5: KINDS OF NGO BUSINESS COLLABORATION

Fund Raising	6
Public Education	5
Training of Business	3
Training of NGOs	1
Publicity for Business	5

TABLE 6: PREPARATION UNDERTAKEN TO INITIATE CONTACT WITH THE BUSINESS SECTOR

Program Development	7
Analysis of Business Policies regarding support of social programmes	5
Analysis of Business AIDS policies	6
Research of other NGO Programmes	3
Programme packaging and presentation	3

TABLE 7: BARRIERS ENCOUNTERED IN WORKING WITH THE BUSINESS SECTOR

AIDS as a Topic	
Management receptivity	6
Worker receptivity	4
Ignorance/Denial of relevance of AIDS	5
Different Expectations/ Corporate Cultures	1
Poor Management of NGO resources/over-extending	3
Lack: of NGO knowledge and skills regarding business	3

TABLE 8: FACTORS TO SUCCESSFUL NGO/BUSINESS RELATIONSHIP	
Credibility of NGO	7
Recognizing mutual benefits	7
Clear focus of collaboration	6
Good follow-up	7

LEARNING POINTS

1. The main barriers to working with business are:
   - incompatibility between the goals and work styles of NGOs and businesses;
   - the relative lack of management and planning skills on the part of NGOs.
2. Although NGOs generally do not think of the business sector as an ally, the business sector can be effective partner and assist NGOs to attain their goals.
3. Assistance from businesses can come in many forms; not only funding, but also technical support, e.g., graphic design and printing, English language skills, accounting and management skills and other in-kind services.
4. In general, HIV and AIDS are new issues for NGOs and business alike.
5. NGOs should approach the business sector as a partner, not just as a potential source of funds, and initiate discussion in order to define areas of common interest and benefit.
6. The NGOs must know the companies with whom they are working. In order to develop a successful partnership with a business, the NGO should have a specific project to present to a business which defines activities and responsibilities of both parties. This proposal should include a justification which reflects the NGO's understanding of the needs of businesses.
7. NGOs should encourage businesses to adopt non-discriminatory policies toward people living with HIV as part of any activities which are conducted jointly with business.
8. A caution was raised that perhaps too much attention is paid to business sector's "bottom line". NGOs also have a "bottom line". Programmes and projects should be developed which will benefit both partners.
9. Personal contacts and friendship building are an absolute necessity. The best contact point is the person at the top of the company- the President or Vice-President

responsible for Human Resources- as s/he is in a decision making position.

10. It is important for NGOs to have a professional image in order to gain access to the business sector. Having business sector representatives on the NGOs' Executive Board can help.

15

Characteristics of Partnerships: The Business Perspective

BILL TIMMERMAN
Deputy Managing Director
Saatchi and Saatchi Advertising
Singapore

1. WHY SHOULD NGO'S WORK WITH THE BUSINESS SECTOR?

It may help them to expand their resource base. It may provide them with a means of expanding their outreach activities.

2. WHAT COULD BE HAPPENING?

Private business could provide the NGO with:

- Funding;
- Sponsorship;
- Use of facilities,
- Volunteer assistance (manpower);
- Etc.

The NGO could be providing business with:

- Employee education and training;
- Counselling on AIDS policy;
- Workplace counselling and services;

3. WHAT'S PREVENTING THIS FROM HAPPENING?

Obstacles for Business:

Businesses do not see the need to get involved. Typical quotes included:

"The problem hasn't surfaced here yet";

"It's the government's job".

The business may not want to be associated with something "negative".

The business worries about "negative Public Relations".

The Priority is "bottom line"; little or no funds for "community relations".

If funds are available, competition from other "causes".

Obstades for NGOS:

Not in a position to offer services or resources. Lac} of wcontacts". Not experienced in dealing with private business.

4. WHAT DOES TOP MANAGEMENT SAY ABOUT WORKING WITH HIV/AIDS RELATED NGOS?

The approach should be to the top.

A direct approach is better than going through business associations.

Any involvement must result in benefit to the business.

Direct benefits are not credible. There will always be better ways to improve bottom line.

The appeal can more compelling if linked to the broad corporate objectives of the business.

5. CORPORATE OBJECTIVES

"....to be a social, economic and intellectual asset to the community in which we operate".

6. WHAT DOES TOP MANAGEMENT SAY ABOUT THE POTENTIAL BENEFIT OF WORKING WITH HIV/AIDS RELATED NGOS?

"If done in the proper way, championing this issue, which until not too long ago was not seen in the best possible light, can improve the image of the company."

7. HOW IS AIDS DIFFERENT?

Education and knowledge —change of behavior is the only weapon. The high degree of direct control an individual can exercise over the amount of risk. At this point, a businessman can do more than a hospital.

SUMMARY POINTS

Know the business, watch the newspapers for information about businesses which you plan to target.

Do not be shy about approaching business - they want help and want to help. Go to the top and go direct.

Analyse the company before you talk to its members. Find out about its corporate objectives and corporate culture.

Find out what experience it has already had with HIV/AIDS related NGOs or with AIDS issues.

Act and look professional.

Start small, be patient, but keep the momentum going.

SURVEY RESULTS

	Electronics Industry	Hotel Indlistry
Does AIDS have an impact on your business?	MOST: "No problem yet" SOME: Yes, but only as part of the larger health education programme.	MOST: No, not at the moment; too early to tell ONE: Yes
What have you done?	Education, counselling	SOME: Talks by Ministry of Health SOME: Nothing
Are you aware of a local NGO (AIDS related)?	No	MOST: Yes SOME: No
What HIV/AIDS related services do you require?	ALL: Counselling support; policy guidance SOME: Legal advice, training, counselling support.	MOST: Training/ education SOME: Legal advice, policy guidance

LEARNING POINTS

1. NGOs' appeal to business is most likely to be compelling if linked to the broad corporate objectives of the business.
2. Businesses are aware that there will be an increase in operating costs as a result of HIV and AIDS. The health

and well being of employees and clients/consumers is a concern of any profit making organization.

3. Businesses are all different. NGOs should understand the nature of the business and its corporate objectives prior to approaching a business.
4. Business will need to be selective in choosing their NGO partners. Therefore, it is vital that businesses have access to information about individual NGOs and the services which they provide.
5. While a connection with AIDS awareness is no longer negative for most businesses, many will still avoid being associated with controversial programs, e.g., providing condoms to sex workers or needles to injecting drug users.
6. NGOs should try to relate directly to senior executives with decision making authority. Trade associations and service organizations, (e.g., Lions, Rotary, Chambers of Commerce) can often assist NGOs to develop these contacts.
7. National NGO councils or coalitions may lend credibility to NGOs and thereby assist individual NGOs to gain access to senior management.
8. NGOs should bring specific proposals for collaboration to businesses. This will help the business develop a sense of "ownership" of a project or cause, e.g., the Worldwide Fund for Nature now fund raises successfully in this manner.

•••